PERMANENT
WEIGHT CONTROL

PERMANENT
WEIGHT CONTROL

MICHAEL J. MAHONEY, Ph.D.
KATHRYN MAHONEY, M.S.W., M.S.

Foreword by Henry A. Jordan, M.D.
Co-Director, Behavioral Weight Control Program
University of Pennsylvania

W·W·NORTON & COMPANY, INC· New York

First Edition

Library of Congress Cataloging in Publication Data

Mahoney, Michael J
  Permanent weight control.

  Bibliography: p.
  Includes index.
  1. Reducing.   2. Corpulence—Psychological aspects.
3. Food habits.   I. Mahoney, Kathryn, joint author.
II. Title.
RC628.M34 1976   616.3'98'0019   75–37739
ISBN 0–393–08736–0

Published simultaneously in Canada
by George J. McLeod Limited, Toronto

Printed in the United States of America

1 2 3 4 5 6 7 8 9

To our families,
and our friends who are like family —
Lynn and Freda, Bobby and Carole.

Contents

Foreword

A simple prescription for loss of weight has been known for centuries—reduce food intake and increase physical activity. Brillat-Savarin, the famous French gourmet and author, in 1825 stated: "Any cure for obesity must begin with the three following and absolute precepts: discretion in eating, moderation in sleeping, and exercise on foot and horseback." This is indeed good advice and has been the foundation for many weight reduction schemes devised over the years. Recently, because of our society's excessive concern for thinness, countless dietary, exercise, and psychological approaches have been advanced, each expounding its virtues and successes in the treatment of obesity. Despite the remarkable claims based on weight loss in a few individuals, these treatments have failed to produce the ultimate goal: permanent weight loss.

Stop-gap measures and partial successes are indeed frustrating to the dieter, and they result from a failure to realize that being overweight is influenced by many aspects of one's life. In our society, for example, the great abundance of attractive, highly palatable foods and the great reliance on labor-saving devices lead most of us to overeat and underexercise.

It is with this knowledge that Michael and Kathryn Mahoney have produced this remarkable book, a book which must be considered a major advance in the treatment of weight problems. The Mahoneys will teach you how to be your own personal scientist, how to analyze your own behaviors, attitudes, and personal thoughts. Once you can understand the factors that influence your behaviors and thoughts you are in a position to make the necessary changes. The Mahoneys are not offering magic nor promising any miracles, but are providing you with the necessary tools to produce gradual, permanent weight loss.

This is not simply a "do" or "don't" book, but rather a book directed at helping you to learn about yourself. It is based on principles derived from the careful work of scores of researchers who have studied the behavior and attitudes of overweight individuals. The major thrust of the book is to help you explore your patterns of behavior and thought, to experiment with change, to test consequences, and to incorporate new behaviors and thoughts into your everyday life. In successive steps, the book examines the major problems—eating, activity, and personal attitude—and provides solutions for their control through a learned process of self-management. The Mahoneys have pioneered an approach that successfully combines two distinct but complementary techniques: behavior change and attitude change. Their book is a milestone because it is the first to apply this comprehensive method to the treatment of overweight individuals.

We are greatly indebted to the Mahoneys for providing this step forward. It is a book that you will turn to again and again as new problems arise and you become interested in understanding and changing your thoughts, attitudes, and behaviors. Successful weight reduction and maintenance is no easy task, but this book will provide the necessary educative steps and techniques for those who are willing to become their own personal scientist.

Henry A. Jordan, M.D.
Co-Director, Behavioral Weight
Control Program,
University Of Pennsylvania

PERMANENT
WEIGHT CONTROL

1
This Can Be the Last Reducing Program of Your Life

If you are like most dieters, this isn't the first book you have read about reducing. As a matter of fact, you may have a large home library of calorie guides, tasteless recipes, and an assortment of best sellers that promise overnight success. You have probably suffered through mounds of cottage cheese and fish and perhaps nearly drowned in ice water and diet soda. For some of you, the ordeal was a total failure. After a few days of religious devotion to hard-boiled eggs and bouillon, you said, "The heck with it—I'd rather be fat than miserable!" Others of you may have stuck to the Spartan diet for several weeks. Some pounds departed—maybe as many as five in a week— and you felt good about your success. The more confident you felt, the more you "eased up." After all, you lost 15 pounds, didn't you? Gradually, you drifted back to your old eating patterns and—just as gradually—your hard-lost pounds reappeared (sometimes bringing a few extra back with them).

This sad series of events is all too common. It is sometimes called the "yo-yo" pattern—going through a never-ending cycle of feast and famine. Nutritionist Jean Mayer of Harvard calls it the "rhythm method of girth control." During years of patient reducing, an individual may gain and lose the same pounds several times over before he finally decides that it's just no use.

Temporary diets—the kind that last for a few weeks and drastically limit the foods you are allowed to eat—almost always fail. You can lose weight with them, sure, but unless they are nutritionally balanced and "easy to get along with," they will go the way of many other good intentions. It is sad that so many motivated and serious weight watchers spend a tremendous amount of time and personal sacrifice in sticking to a special diet, only to become discouraged when

3

they drift back to their original eating and exercise habits, which were the real culprits in the first place. By focusing their efforts on changing general styles of eating and activity, these people could have achieved more permanent and rewarding weight reduction.

The yo-yo cycle is not only discouraging, but it may be much more dangerous to your health than staying overweight. Recent medical evidence has questioned the advisability of popular "quick loss" diets, which result in a temporary reduction followed by a quick rebound. This is because much of the structural damage done to the heart and arteries in obesity seems to occur during weight *gain*. Thus, *a person who continually reduces and regains may be placing more of a strain on his heart than one who maintains a relatively constant number of excess pounds!* The important point here, of course, is that a truly successful reducing program should have lasting effects. If you can't lose weight comfortably with a program that is easy enough to live with for the rest of your life, then you might be better off not trying to reduce at all. Don't misunderstand—excess pounds *are* a known hazard to your health. You're taking a risk with your personal well-being each day that you carry around that extra weight (the more pounds, the greater the risk). However, the health risk of losing and then regaining may be even more dangerous. Obviously, having your choice between two serious threats to your life and happiness is not an enviable position. It would be nice to have a third, low risk option— namely, losing those dangerous excess pounds without running the high risk of regaining them. This book is devoted to giving you that option. It is designed to help you lose weight *permanently*. That's right, permanently. Assuming that you read on and utilize the self-control techniques that are described, *this can be your last reducing program!*

Now then, what makes this book so special? Why should it help you lose permanently when nothing else has? Those are fair questions. The defense rests on two points:

1. The approach outlined in this book is geared toward permanence. You aren't asked to go "on" a diet or exercise program because going "on" a diet means that someday you'll go "off" it. You wouldn't consent to eating only cottage

cheese and hard-boiled eggs for the rest of your life, would you? Of course not! Then why start? Can you honestly say you'll never eat another doughnut? Then why begin a diet that is doomed to be broken? Popular diets restrict your eating. Not only does this make the forbidden foods more tempting, but it also sets up an unreasonable goal of perfection. Your first sweet or bad day "blows the diet" and you give up. *There are no forbidden foods or compulsory calisthenics in the program presented in this book.* Does that mean you can eat whatever you want? In one sense, yes. It is recommended that you allow yourself an occasional dessert or high calorie meal. To do this and still lose weight, of course, you have to make room for these calories elsewhere. Notice that you're working on an overall balance, allowing yourself some acceptable treats by developing general eating patterns that can accommodate them without weight gain. The rule of thumb here is: IF YOU CAN'T LIVE WITH IT, DON'T START IT. That means, of course, that the techniques which are recommended will be relatively easy and very gradual. You won't lose five pounds per week, but you will have the satisfaction of knowing that the pounds you lose can be gone forever.

2. The second defense is evidence. Over 50 scientific experiments involving more than 2000 obese individuals have supported the superiority of the type of approach presented here. Although there is still much room for improvement, the techniques presented in this book represent the most effective scientifically tested means now available for permanent weight control.

If you are disgusted with your previous temporary losses and if the prospect of never again "dieting" sounds inviting, this program should appeal to you. At this time next year it will be a pleasant change not to be facing that perennial "battle of the bulge." Imagine how nice it will be to control your weight without the agony of continual dieting! You can be a healthier, happier, and thinner person without starving yourself or suffering through mounds of cottage cheese and years of aerobics. By developing comfortable and livable eating and activity styles with the techniques described in this book, you can solve your weight problem once and for all.

Lasting weight loss, of course, is not something you achieve overnight. If you are searching for a magical and effortless solution to your weight problem, modern science has little to offer you. There are dozens of best sellers that promise you immediate and substantial losses. However, the honesty of their claims is questionable, particularly if you want to keep the weight off. One of the most appealing aspects of this program is its supporting evidence. You are not going to be given a Madison Avenue pitch. No wild claims for effortless overnight success will be made. However, an optimism based on the findings of controlled scientific research will be shared. But, you might argue, every other reducing book also claims extensive supporting evidence. The author usually has an M.D. or a Ph.D. and assures you that his own clinical records attest to the miracle-working powers of his new diet. How is our program any different? Well, aside from offering cautious optimism rather than religious fervor, we are providing you with the technical references that will allow you to evaluate the evidence for yourself. You need not take our word for it—the research articles speak for themselves. The consumer is well advised to be skeptical of the many ambitious claims made about weight reduction. Americans spend millions of dollars per year on dietary aids. The "fight fat" business has been a lucrative market for authors and (ironically) food producers. Unfortunately, the overweight American seems to swallow unresearched reducing schemes with almost as much ease as he swallows his breakfast doughnut. If a weight loss book is authored by someone with initials after his name, it is accepted as dietary gospel. If the author describes a handful of dramatically successful case histories, all possibility for doubt is removed. The enthusiastic weight watcher buys the book and races home to begin his miraculous transformation into a gaunt and sexy new person. When that new person fails to materialize, the undaunted dieter simply searches for another miracle-working program.

It is sad but true that many of the popular weight loss books have little or no formal scientific research supporting their effectiveness. Their only claims to success are often the clinical records of their authors, and authors seldom report their failures. After all, failures don't sell books. The unsuspecting reader is, therefore, forced to trust the author's statements about "extensive medical evidence" and clinical successes. Judging from recent investigations and nutritional evaluations of popular reducing programs, that trust has been sorely abused. Not only have some of these programs shown very poor results in producing permanent weight loss, but several have been shown to be potentially dangerous to the health of the reducer.

The claims made in this book do not presume your trust. In fact, they invite your skepticism. It is only through doubting that you will test, and it is only through testing that you will learn whether the program presented here can be beneficial to you. Test the scientific evidence. Consult the technical articles listed in the References. Notice that their results are not miracles—but generally positive. The real tests, of course, is not whether thousands of people have benefited from this kind of program. The critical test is whether this book offers strategies that can help *you* with your weight problem. And that test is again one which we welcome with cautious optimism.

If you are a skeptic about all the promises and cure-alls that have flooded the reducing market, this program is well suited to you. It promises to give you returns equal only to your investments. That is, it doesn't deny that enduring weight loss takes time and conscientious effort. However, the evidence has demonstrated that permanent weight control *is* possible and that it does not require unreasonable effort or perpetual hunger.

This book is intended to provide you with some helpful suggestions on how to develop a permanently successful reducing program. Three major elements are emphasized: (1) your motivation and commitment to long-term self-improvement, (2) accurate knowledge about the causes and solution of weight problems, and (3) personal adoption of effective techniques to change eating and exercise habits. This book presents technical information and guidelines for your development of self-control skills. You will learn about the *role of thinking in weight loss* and *the importance of encouragement from family and friends.* A brief discussion of *nutrition* will indicate the dangers of many popular fad diets and suggest methods for making your daily eating both more nutritious and less fattening. You will learn about *the importance of physical activity* in successful reducing, and many old myths will be challenged. Finally, you will learn about *the psychology of eating*—

why sweets are so rewarding and vacations so fattening, and why some people eat because of boredom or "nervous energy." The critical importance of *maintaining your motivation* will also be discussed.

In addition to this technical information, you will receive step-by-step instructions on how to do it—where to start, how to enlist the support of family and friends, how to reduce sensibly and nutritiously. You will learn ways to change *what* you eat, *where* and *when* you eat, *how* you eat, and *why* you eat. Techniques for increasing your physical activity without unreasonable calisthenics will be presented, along with effective strategies for handling tension and boredom eating. Perhaps most important, you will receive suggestions on how to maintain your motivation and your progress so that this is, indeed, *the last reducing program of your life.*

2
Reduction Readiness

It takes more than motivation and effort to reduce successfully—your attitudes and knowledge play an important role. Unfortunately, the area of weight control is overrun with myths and misconceptions. Many self-proclaimed experts offer their pet theories about who can reduce, the most successful methods for reducing, and so on. The determined weight watcher seldom challenges these myths, and they often get in the way of more reasonable or effective self-control. For example, did you know that *each of the following statements is false?*

SOME POPULAR MISCONCEPTIONS ABOUT REDUCING

1. *Most weight problems are inherited.* Although there is some evidence for inherited aspects of body frame and size, excess fat is not transmitted through the genes—it must be acquired through an energy imbalance. Individuals do vary, of course, in their daily caloric needs and in their tendency to accumulate or eliminate excess fat—but these differences do not contradict the fact that calories consumed must exceed calories spent for a person to become fat.

2. *A person whose parents were overweight or who has been obese since childhood is probably "naturally fat."* This statement, like the preceding one, is far from accurate. The fact that obesity often runs in families and sometimes begins early in life is at least partially due to the fact that children acquire many of their eating and activity habits from their parents.

3. *Hormone problems—particularly thyroid deficiencies—are responsible for many cases of obesity.* Although this statement was once believed by health professionals, recent evidence suggests that a very, very small percentage of weight problems is influenced by hormone imbalances. Even in those very rare cases where hormone imbalance may be a factor, however, you are not doomed to permanent obesity. With proper medication and appropriate adjustments in your energy balance, you can reduce successfully.

4. *Exercise isn't a very useful way to reduce—it doesn't burn many calories and it just makes a person hungrier.* As we shall see in a later chapter, this statement couldn't be farther from the truth. Moderate increases in personal activity patterns can make a tremendous difference in the rate and maintenance of weight loss. Moreover, moderate amounts of exercise actually make you less hungry than if you were very inactive.

5. *Eliminating all fats and carbohydrates is the quickest way to reduce.* Absolutely not! A diet that contains no fats at all actually slows down the rate of weight loss. Moreover, fat-free and carbohydrate-free diets endanger your health.

6. *It is impossible to reduce by eating health foods.* This is again a very serious misrepresentation. Some currently popular health foods (e.g., granola, yogurt, and wheat germ) are, indeed, high in calories. However, there are a number of ways you can include these foods in a reasonable reducing program.

7. *Drugs are often helpful in reducing.* False! Investigations of the effectiveness of prescription reducing drugs (usually amphetamines, thyroid extracts, or appetite suppressants) suggest that they have little if any effect on long-term weight control. The same is true for over-the-counter reducing aids, diuretics, and laxatives. Some individuals may lose initially, but months later they have regained the weight (and sometimes added a little extra).

8. *Obesity is a symptom of deep personality problems, and its successful treatment requires prolonged psychotherapy to get at the real cause.* This popular myth has probably been responsible for more misery and fear than any other. Judging from the available scientific evidence, however, it is false. Although many poor eating habits are learned early in life (e.g., "clean up your plate," "sweets are treats"), they can be changed successfully without psychotherapy. Overeating is not a symptom of mental disturbance. More reasonable eating and exercise habits can be learned, whether you are 20 or 70, and regardless of how many previous dieting failures you have had.

9. *Weighing yourself every day is an aid to reducing.* Wrong. Permanent losses are not seen on the scales every 24 hours. The average home scale is not accurate enough to detect the small but reasonable daily losses that occur in an enduring weight loss program. Besides, fluctuation in water retention and colon activity may result in temporary gains or "plateaus." If your motivation is riding on a daily weigh-in, you can expect to be disappointed. Therefore, don't weigh yourself more than once every two weeks.

10. *It is normal to gain weight as you get older.* There is nothing normal or natural about getting fat. The middle-aged spread is not inevitable—it is usually the result of gradual reductions in physical activity without corresponding reductions in calorie intake. Even though the food needs of the average adult decline each year, he or she often continues eating the same types and quantities of food that were appropriate for an active and growing young person.

11. *A person who is not successful at reducing often lacks will power.* This kind of argument is a familiar and perhaps comforting one to the unsuccessful weight watcher. It is easy to excuse failure on the basis of some mysterious inner force. However, recent evidence has shown that self-control is *not* an inborn strength which some people possess and others lack. The successful reducer does not owe his success to some inherited personality trait. Self-control is now known to be a complex but learnable set of personal skills. But, you may ask, why do some people reduce so easily while others—perhaps including yourself—have failed repeatedly? The difference is not one of will power. Although age, activity, and metabolism play an important part, the major difference lies in learnable skills. Regardless of your age, your past history of failures, or your degree of obesity, you *can* learn to control your weight effectively and permanently.

Did any of the above myths or attitudes sound familiar? Let's briefly discuss some of the general facts about obesity and reducing.

WHAT IS OBESITY?

Obesity is a condition involving excessive fat (adipose tissue). In small quantities, fat is very useful as a source of stored energy and as a body insulator. It is also an element in the storage and absorption of some vitamins (A, D, E, and K). However, excessive fat tissue may pose serious problems.

To specify the degree of obesity of a particular individual, you are frequently referred to a standardized weight table. Unfortunately, most of the publicly available weight tables list American averages—which do not take into account the fact that the average American is overweight. Some tables of desirable bodyweights have been developed to remedy this problem. Unfortunately, height-weight tables are not very accurate or useful in judging degree of obesity. This is because *your bodyweight is not a very accurate measure of your body fat.* That's right! Many things other than fat accumulation affect your weight—muscle size, water retention, bone structure, and so on. A healthy football player may be heavier than what is often considered desirable for his height, but his extra pounds are probably extra muscles rather than fat.

There are some very accurate methods for measuring bodyfat, but most of them require technical instruments. For example, skinfold thickness is a very good index of obesity. Place your thumb and index finger about an inch apart on your cheek and squeeze them gently together. The thickness of your folded cheek is an indirect measure of your body fat. Approximately half of your total body fat is stored just beneath the skin. When you pinch or fold a small area, you can measure the thickness of the fold and use that as an index of fatness. As a matter of fact, scientists can measure your skinfold thickness with a very precise pinching instrument (called a skinfold caliper) and then give you an accurate estimate of your total body fat. They arrive at this figure by using mathematical equations. Normal, healthy men are often between 10 and 13 percent fat, while the average-weight woman may be as much as 25 percent adipose!

You can estimate your own fat content by measuring the skinfold thickness of your upper arm. Have a friend or family member stand behind you. Your arms should rest at your sides with palms facing inward. The most accurate index of your total fat content is the thickness of your upper arm (triceps) skinfold. On the back side of your right arm, have your helper choose a spot about halfway between your shoulder and your elbow. Ask him to place the tip of his thumb and index finger about one inch apart at that spot on your arm. Now have him pinch up the skin into a fold, making sure to pull the soft fat tissue away from the muscle underneath. (You can check this by flexing your muscle.) With your skin still pinched, ask him to measure the thickness of the fold using a ruler or tape measure. Do this several times on the back of each arm to make sure you have a fairly good estimate. This is, of course, a very rough way of estimating your fat content. However, you can draw some approximate conclusions as follows. If your skinfold thickness is greater than one inch, you probably have a relatively high fat content (or your pinching helper made a mistake). Between half an inch and an inch you still have plenty of room to reduce. Measurements much below half an inch indicate normal or below normal fat content, particularly for men. Remember, this estimate is an approximate one.

Most dieters don't need any additional evidence of their weight problem—tight clothing, a bulging abdomen, and the hard cold facts from their bathroom scale convince them that weight reduction is needed. However, many people like to have a quantified goal in their reduction efforts. This may account for the popularity of height-weight tables. A very approximate "ideal" weight can be determined as follows. For women, multiply your height in inches by 3.5 and then subtract 110. This will give you a fairly accurate estimate of a desira-

$$\text{desirable weight} = (\text{height} \times 3.5) - 110$$
(woman)

ble nude weight. Thus, a woman of five foot four (64 inches) should weigh about 114 pounds. For men, an approximate ideal weight can be determined by multiplying height in inches by 4 and then subtracting 130. A six foot one male should, therefore, weigh about 162

$$\text{desirable weight} = (\text{height} \times 4) - 130$$
(man)

pounds. Remember that these "ideals" do not take many factors, such as muscularity and body frame, into account. They should, therefore, be viewed as very approximate figures.

THE POSITIVE ENERGY CRISIS

One can visualize the human body as a complex system that both requires and spends energy. The energy is measured in calories. Daily tissue repairs, maintaining a constant body temperature, physical activity, fighting infections, and a variety of other bodily functions require caloric energy. This is provided by food intake as well as stored energy sources (fat and glycogen). When the body's energy needs are adequately met without much surplus, a relatively constant state exists—your bodyweight remains stable. If caloric intake is less than current energy needs, a *negative energy crisis* · develops—the body must resort to stored energy sources. (Glycogen and fat are usually broken down first.) If this "fuel shortage" continues over a lengthy period of time, your body will begin digesting your own muscles and organs. As a matter of fact, there is now evidence that *lengthy starvation diets and diets that totally avoid fats or carbohydrates* may pose serious health hazards because they often *result in the breakdown of muscle and organ protein rather than body fat*. This is one reason to avoid eating programs that limit calories to less than 1000 per day or totally eliminate either fats or carbohydrates.

Obesity is caused by a positive energy crisis—the number of calories consumed is greater than the body's current needs. This excess fuel is converted into fat for storage. For every 3500 surplus calories, approximately one pound of fat is deposited. These surplus calories need not come from rich or sweet foods—excess protein calories are also converted to fat. Thus, the person who eats "good" dietetic foods and yet fails to reduce may still be consuming too many calories. The energy imbalance in obesity can be corrected by (1) reducing the number of calories consumed, (2) increasing bodily energy requirements (through exercise, for example), or (3) both of the above.

WHAT'S A LITTLE FAT GOING TO HURT?

Your reason for wanting to reduce can play an important role in your success. For many dieters, weight control is a cosmetic pursuit—that is, they want to look more attractive. There is, of course, nothing wrong with desiring a healthy, trim figure. However, fair weather motivation—the kind that comes right after the holidays and just before the beaches open—lasts for only a couple of weeks. Temporary reasons produce temporary results.

If your motivation to reduce is based on concern for personal health and well-being, however, chances are that you will be willing to invest a little more effort. But how much of a health risk is involved in obesity? After all, you can probably think of people you know who are overweight and yet apparently healthy. They may even be elderly. Is excess fat *always* bad for you?

The simplest answer is "No." There are some mildly and moderately obese persons whose health is not conspicuously threatened by their excess pounds. There are, in fact, some times when you might be advised not to reduce (for example, during pregnancy or if ulcerative colitis, regional ileitis, or Addison's disease is suspected). However, the general relationship between obesity and health is unquestionable: *excess fat poses a serious health problem.* The risk involved generally increases with age. Also, the greater the degree of obesity, the greater the risk.

What kinds of health risks are we talking about? Many of you may already be aware of the known relationship between obesity and heart attacks. The risk of heart disease is tremendously increased in moderately and extremely overweight individuals. For example, when compared with persons of normal weight, the obese suffer about one and a half times more heart diseases. As a matter of fact, a wide range of serious health hazards has been shown to occur more frequently among obese individuals. Many of these disorders are related to one another and work together to present a critical threat to your health and happiness.

The following conditions are often associated with or complicated by obesity:

1. Diseases of the heart and arteries
   a. arteriosclerosis (hardening of the arteries)
   b. heart enlargement
   c. hypertension (high blood pressure)
   d. angina pectoris
   e. brain hemorrhage
   f. varicose veins
   g. congestive heart failure
   h. reactive polycythemia (increased red blood count)
2. Diabetes
3. Cirrhosis of the liver
4. Appendicitis

5. Other disorders
   a. kidney diseases
   b. the Pickwickian syndrome (constant fatigue often associated with shortness of breath and ruddy cheeks)
   c. toxemia of pregnancy, difficult deliveries
   d. arthritis
   e. surgical complications
   f. breathing difficulties

Although it is sometimes impossible to know whether obesity causes each of the above conditions, there is good reason to believe that sensible and permanent weight reduction lowers the risk of suffering from them.

Let's take a second here to review some of the reasons for reducing. In addition to improving physical appearance, permanent weight loss can dramatically reduce the risk of heart disease. It can add years to your life as well as increase your ability to enjoy those extra years. Enduring weight loss can improve physical endurance, reduce fatigue, and lower the risk of diabetes and other serious diseases. It can help to improve breathing problems and reduce the likelihood of surgical complications. Added to all of these personal advantages are several that are frequently overlooked. The successful reducer is often a healthier and happier companion—a more active parent and a more valued spouse. In addition to increasing the amount and quality of healthy companionship for his or her family, the persevering weight watcher sets a valuable example for both friends and family. He is tackling a difficult personal problem with patient persistence and a dedication to lasting self-improvement.

You now have a choice—perhaps the most important choice of your life. Sure, you've decided to diet before, and maybe it has almost become a joking matter. But think for a second about the facts we have just reviewed. Obesity is a serious threat to your daily happiness and your very life. If you would like to have a little more time and a lot more ability to do things in your life—if adding some extra healthy years to share with your loved ones is appealing, then you have a choice to make. You are now beginning a program that has been very effective in helping people reduce. Its effectiveness, however, is not magical. It must be given sincere effort. The technical knowledge and how-to-do-it suggestions will be helpful only if you use them. The choice is yours—you can decide that it's not worth it and face the perennial risks of your poor physical condition, *or* you can choose to start on the last reducing program of your life.

3
Thick and Thin:
What Makes the Difference?

Regardless of your age, sex, or heredity, if you are overweight, you are overfueled. Your body's needs for energy are not only being met—they are being exceeded, and you are carrying around this surplus energy in the form of fat. The solution for getting rid of that excess can be stated very simply: CHANGE YOUR INTAKE OR OUTPUT OF ENERGY. Ideally, both of these options should be pursued. You should work not only on reducing calorie intake, but also on increasing the amount of energy you spend in everyday activities.

Simple, right? Then why is obesity such a widespread problem? Why don't more people simply correct their energy imbalance and live happily and thinly ever after? More important, why is it that some people seem to be able to lose weight so easily while others struggle for months with no progress? Aren't there chemical, genetic, or psychological factors that make the difference?

As we saw in the last chapter, these factors are frequently offered to explain or excuse weight loss failure. The conscientious dieter may suffer through weeks of Spartan semistarvation, only to lose less than a pound. Ironically, he or she often has a friend who seems immune to obesity. These fortunate beanpoles seem to eat everything in sight and never gain a pound. They often brag that when they want to lose weight they just "make up their minds" and magically shed 10 or 20 pounds. Surely, there must be some striking differences between the perpetual pudge and the sweet-eating skeleton? Let's discuss some of the possibilities.

GENETICS

Could the overweight person have inherited his or her problem? Very, very unlikely. The genetic transmission of obesity in humans is re-

18

stricted to a few diseases (e.g., the Laurence-Moon-Biedl syndrome), which are so rare that they are hardly worth considering. But, you might argue, many overweight people have obese parents, while thin people frequently come from thin families. This is true. However, the fact that something "runs in families" does not necessarily mean that it is inherited. Children often imitate their parents' lifestyles. Thin parents may thus set an example of balanced eating and a reasonable activity level. Notice the implications of this for your own reducing efforts. To the extent that you "model" a commitment to personal growth and self-improvement, you may provide your own children with a valuable example of life-saving skills. By observing your efforts to resolve a difficult personal problem, they may learn both values and skills that will be beneficial to their own later happiness.

Before considering another possible factor, it should be mentioned that heredity is not totally irrelevant to reducing. Although you may not have inherited fat, you did inherit a body frame, and there is some evidence that body frame may make a difference in obesity. The petite skeleton—characterized by generally smaller bone structure and less muscularity—seems less inclined to accumulate fat. The "inclination" here is not a violation of the energy balance concept; it simply states that people with slighter frames tend to be lighter. This may be the result of increased activity, decreased food intake, or both. A word of caution here—it is easy to conclude that since you are overweight, you *must* have a large frame. Not so. It is very difficult to estimate body frame dimensions from simple visual inspection. Precise measurements of hip girth, bone mass, muscle density, and wrist and ankle size are required to evaluate body frame accurately. But, for the sake of argument, let's assume that you do indeed have a moderate or large skeletal frame. Are you therefore doomed to a life of chronic obesity? Absolutely not. You are still a prime candidate for successful weight loss, but with one qualification. Your ultimate goal in weight reduction should not be unreasonable. Although you can effectively improve your health and appearance, it may be unlikely that you will attain the svelte proportions of a Twiggy. No amount of reducing or plastic surgery can change your body frame. You will simply have to accept the fact that you have a somewhat larger or more muscular frame than some of your movie idols. While weight reduction may not be able to make you a wisp of a person, however, it can still prolong your life, improve your appearance, and add to the happiness you share with your friends and family.

METABOLISM

Okay, so the difference between the perpetual pudge and the sweet-eating skeleton is probably not genetic. Could it be metabolic? Maybe the thin person burns fat faster or converts less of his food to adipose? Possibly, but again with qualifications. "Metabolism" is a summary term for the chemical processes involved in energy regulation. Individuals may vary in the speed and efficiency of these processes. The energy balance that is so important in obesity is unavoidably influenced by metabolism. Individuals with higher metabolic rates are less likely to gain weight than persons with lower rates. Is that your problem? Are your "fat burners" slower or less efficient than other people's? First of all, the evidence for gross metabolic differences between obese and nonobese people is very rare. The popular belief that most overweight people suffer from a thyroid deficiency (hypothyroidism) is a stubborn myth that seems to persist despite medical evidence to the contrary. A dieter need only hear about one or two cases of hypothyroid obesity to maintain his or her belief that his or her own weight problem stems from a similar cause. Unfortunately, many physicians prescribe thyroid medication without an actual laboratory test to determine deficiency.[1] The fact that there are not *gross* differences in metabolism between normal and overweight people, however, does not necessarily mean that there may not be *any* differences. Recent medical evidence has suggested, for example, that individuals may vary slightly in the arithmetic of their weight reduction. On the average, 3500 calories constitute a pound. For some individuals, however, this figure may vary by as much as several hundred calories. While a surplus of nearly 4000 calories may be needed for the thin person to gain a pound, the chronic weight watcher may require as little as 3000 surplus calories. If each of these individuals consumes an extra 100 calories per day for a year, the thinner person will gain 9.1 pounds and the second will be 12.2 pounds heavier. While this dif-

---

[1] An analysis of serum thyroxine can be performed very easily with a blood sample. Normal values are 4 to 11 micrograms per 100 milliliters (total) and 0.8 to 2.4 millimicrograms per 100 milliliters (free).

ference is certainly not insignificant, it is also insufficient to explain gross obesity. Notice that this metabolic factor does not *cause* a weight problem. It can only *contribute* by allowing some persons less tolerance for surplus calories. With the judicious reduction of only 100 calories per day, our fatter friend in the above example could have ended the year without any weight gain.

While on this topic, the recent evidence on infantile obesity should perhaps be discussed. Although the data are still very preliminary, there is some indication that weight problems that began in childhood may leave an indelible mark on the individual's body composition. According to one theory recently suggested, people who have been fat since infancy may encounter more difficulties in reducing than people whose weight problems began later in life. The theoretical rationale goes as follows. A person can get fat in one of two ways—by increasing his number of fat cells (adipocytes) or by increasing the size of already existing cells. Recent research has suggested that an overfed infant or child stores surplus calories by increasing cell number. Sometime around adolescence, the body stops building new fat cells and begins storing excess calories by simply enlarging existing fat cells. This means that the childhood-onset obese person may have many more fat cells than the adult-onset person. During weight reduction, the body empties fat deposits but does not actually destroy the cells. Thus two weight watchers may each lose 20 pounds, but if one of them had been fat during childhood, he or she would still have an excess quantity of fat cells. Theoretically, a person's inclination to gain or regain weight may be greater when cell number has been increased. Thus, the childhood-onset dieter's progress may be slower and more unstable than that of his or her friend. These speculations, however, should be viewed very cautiously. The existing research is still far from sufficient, and some recent studies have been reported that childhood-onset obese persons may not be any less successful than others in their reducing. Moreover, even if the theory survives, its implications are again very relative. The early-onset dieter would not be doomed to a life of obesity but only to a more difficult task in permanent reduction. The question of energy balance reigns supreme regardless of differences in arithmetic.

It is therefore unlikely that metabolic or cellular factors make the difference between our perpetual dieter and the eat-anything beanpole. Although these influences can contribute to weight problems by imposing different physiological restrictions on people, they are not sufficient to account for the fat-thin distinction.

PSYCHOLOGICAL

Perhaps the difference is psychological. Maybe the scarecrow has substantially more will power than his corpulent friend? As we saw in the last chapter, this attempted explanation is contradicted by contemporary knowledge about self-control. People are not born with varying quantities of some mysterious inner strenth. It turns out that our language may have played tricks with us in this area. We often say that so-and-so has a lot of will power, meaning that he or she has successfully endured or conquered some formidable problem. In this sense of the term, "will power" means "has shown self-control." Unfortunately, the distinction between *having* and *doing* often gets blurred, so that the person who has done something difficult is frequently said to possess some inner capacity.

But surely we are not saying such things as motivation don't count? Of course not. Motivation is a very important element in successful self-control. However, people are not born with varying quantities of motivation. It isn't some magical force showered on a fortunate few and denied the majority. People frequently talk about their motivation as if it were an unchangeable inner material. Somewhere wedged between their spleen and their kidneys lies this mysterious substance called motivation, and it is presumed to be the source of many valuable abilities. Either you have it or you don't; and if you don't, forget it—yours is a lost cause. This doomsday thinking goes on in all too many heads and is probably responsible for a large percentage of unattempted and quickly terminated self-control efforts.

But if motivation isn't a psychological force, what is it? A technical answer to this question would take more time and effort than we can here afford. Briefly stated, a person's motivation to control his own behavior seems to be a combination of several different factors. Among the most important are (1) the value of the ancitipated change (e.g., health, personal appearance, social desirability, etc.), and (2) his confidence in the feasibility of his control. If the person values some change highly and is confident that the change can be produced, his motivation is usually very high. Interestingly, one of the most important factors in personal motivation seems to be what the person says to himself. A dieter can influence his motivation dramatically simply by changing the content of his private monologues—those intimate conversations he has with himself. Thus, someone who is continually thinking, "This will never work" can, in fact, reduce his own motivation to try. In a later chapter we will talk more about this aspect of self-control. For the time being, let us agree that motivation is an important but adjustable factor in successful weight loss. The fact that a person can exert some influence on his own motivation is a very important one to bear in mind.

We have now surveyed genetic, metabolic, and psychological factors that might account for the difference between an overweight and a normal weight person. Although each area has offered possible influences that could contribute to weight problems, none of them has been sufficient. Obesity is the result of a very complex set of factors. Heredity, metabolism, and motivational influences may be important, but they are apparently not the primary factors. We still haven't accounted for the difference between thick and thin. What is left? Is there any research identifying factors that do separate the obese from the nonobese?

Simply and emphatically: YES. Although our knowledge of the causes of and cures for obesity is still very inadequate, research over the last several decades has suggested some very important factors in understanding weight problems. Much of that knowledge will be summarized in the chapters that follow. By way of preview, however, two important generalizations can be offered.

First, *the major differences between obese and nonobese individuals lie in their eating and activity patterns.* Although physiological and metabolic factors may influence fat mobilization and efficient energy exchange, the primary factors in weight management are the personal habits that affect energy intake and output.

Second, *the major differences between successful and unsuccessful weight watchers lie in their self-control skills.* Will power, heredity, and similar static influences do not account for differential success in reducing. Significant and lasting weight loss is produced by a set of relevant personal skills that help the individual make appropriate changes in his eating and activity patterns.

The significance of these two generalizations can hardly be over-emphasized. They identify both the *sources* of and *solutions* for obesity. It should come as no surprise that the primary culprits in weight problems are food intake and energy expenditure. More interesting, perhaps, is the conclusion that successful reducing requires learnable self-control skills. Knowing *where* the problem lies has little utility unless we also know *how* to attack it.

4
Getting in Focus:
The Culprits Are Patterns,
Not Pounds

Here is a scene that may be familiar to you. It is 3:00 a.m. You are standing in front of the refrigerator, completing your inventory of its cool depths. You scan and bypass the familiar contents of the first shelf—the ever-present diet soda, cottage cheese, and carrot sticks. With a sigh, you shift your gaze to the second shelf and begin your inspection of its more transient contents. Suddenly your eyes light up. Your careful inspection is rewarded. There, on the second shelf, are the remains of that Boston cream pie you served to company for dinner. And you were so good; you didn't even taste it! In fact, you hardly ate a thing and everyone else simply stuffed! With stomach growling and mouth watering, you gaze at it longingly. You can already taste it as you reach for it.

The suddenly you remember that scale upstairs. You glance at the clock. Just four hours until morning and your daily weigh-in. You quickly replay your day. You did so well today; you probably have lost a little. You start to waver. Is it worth it? Should you blow it now? You tear your gaze away from the pie and focus again on the first shelf. You stand silently, lost in thought. After several moments, you reach for a carrot stick and quickly close the door. With a sigh you leave the kitchen, dreading the beginning of another food-dominated day. You go back to bed, comforting yourself with the thought that when those pounds are gone, you will eat all you want, of whatever you want. Then you'll eat Boston cream pie three times a day if you want to. And you'll never touch another carrot stick!

If you can easily see yourself in the leading role of this mental movie, you are well aware of a consistent characteristic of weight watching. You know something every chronic reducer knows. The history of weight watching spans many decades. It has meant different

25

things to different people—various methods, various goals, various standards for "normal" weight. But out of the variety emerges one consistent, even monotonous, theme: *weight control is an effortful endeavor.* Despite claims for effortless losses and overnight successes, it is rarely quick *or* easy. Miracle methods come and go, and standards change. But one feature of weight watching remains the same. Weight control typically takes hard work over a long period of time. It demands dedicated and persistent effort. It is worthwhile, but an effortful, endeavor.

Let's consider your personal memoirs as a weight watcher. If yours are like many others, they may have been written by the light of the refrigerator door! You probably can see yourself in the following scenes: picking at the "low-calorie plate" on your family's night out; sipping bouillon at lunch while your coworkers munch potato chips; sweating in the gym, wishing you were home in bed. And there you are in one of the most familiar of all: gazing into the refrigerator. All those hours! If you lost an ounce for every time you have opened and closed that refrigerator door you'd be a walking skeleton, right?

You probably have an extensive repertoire of scenes like those above to remind you of the effort involved in weight control. You need little convincing of that unwelcome but familiar idea. It may take more to convince you of a second important point: *weight watching, though effortful, can be successful.*

Your individual memoirs may tell a different story. They may reflect months or even years of genuine effort—and still be a sob story! Your autobiography may well be written in terms of *which* diet you were on *when*—and it may still have an unhappy ending. Let's follow up that scene at the refrigerator door. What happened after your "perfect" day? Your memoirs may record several such "perfect days"—days of resolutions kept, temptations resisted, plans followed. They may tell of food-dominated days characterized primarily by resistance, days in which your life literally revolved around food—and your efforts focused mainly on resisting it. Only the veteran dieter knows the true agony of this kind of effort, in which food may become simultaneously the most coveted and the most despised thing in his life. And then, finally, your memoirs report that the resistance has won. You've reached goal weight; your Herculean efforts are rewarded. At last, you are a thinner, more attractive you.

You are ecstatic. Finally, it's all over—no more carrot sticks or calisthenics. You can go off that miserable diet and pack your sweat-suit away. At last, you can eat all those foods you've denied yourself for weeks. At last, you can eat whatever you'd like; you deserve it! And typically, at this point, you'd like plenty. You have made food a prize—to be worked for, earned, and highly valued. You have made it a forbidden fruit. When you finally make those forbidden fruits available to yourself, you are very likely to binge, to gorge yourself with all those self-denied treats you've wanted for so long. At this point the idea of another diet is so aversive that the very thought of it may lead to binge eating. All those days and nights of dieting and here you are again—eating everything in sight as your weight creeps back up. The higher it climbs, the more frustrated you feel—and the more you eat. The frustrations and discouragement resulting from this cycle may seem overwhelming at times. Your personal memoirs may well be entitled, "The Agony and Ecstasy of Weight Watching"—with genuine emphasis on the agony.

If this is your story, it is similar to many others. What is the problem here? How can you devote so much effort, work so hard, and still be unsuccessful? What are the villains in your personal plot that have foiled your efforts and sabotaged your success?

There *are* reasons for your lack of success, and it's important that you understand and remember them. The problem is certainly *not* one of lack of effort, although your failures may have made you question our old proverb: you get out of something what you put into it. Our guideline of "effort equals outcome" may be better expressed: "appropriate effort equals *desired* outcome." If your story ends unhappily, it is probably not the *extent* of your efforts but the *focus* of your efforts that is the problem. You may have fallen prey to the two most basic saboteurs of successful weight control. Stop and review for a moment to see if you can pinpoint them. What are you focusing on that demands such high premiums for low returns?

First, you have probably misfocused on your weight as problem, not product; as source, not side effect. Those excess pounds you carry around constantly remind you of *weight;* it becomes very easy to see your weight as problem, not by-product. Yet, in an important sense, your weight is *not* the problem. As much as you would like to, you cannot manipulate pounds directly. You *can only manipulate pat-*

terns—here's where the real problem lies. As you have already learned, the major difference in obese and nonobese individuals is their eating and exercise patterns. To the extent that pounds distract you from assessing and pinpointing problematical patterns, they are distracting you from *permanent* weight loss and effective weight control.

The second factor follows from the first. If you have misfocused on weight as the source of the problem, you have probably also misfocused on weight loss as the solution. Now, what's wrong with that? After all, if you are overweight successful weight control does include weight loss. But the primary difference between successful and unsuccessful weight watchers lies in their self-control skills. Successful weight watchers are successful self-controllers. They are individuals who concentrate on improving their eating and exercise patterns, not on losing weight. They are more concerned with their eating *habits* than with numbers on the scale. They are justifiably confident that pattern change will *lead* to weight loss and to permanent weight control.

If you have been an unsuccessful weight watcher, your weight watching history probably reveals an overemphasis on weight loss and a lack of emphasis on pattern change. In all likelihood, it describes a frequent result of that overemphasis on weight loss—an exaggeration of the importance of one weight control strategy, namely, caloric restriction. In some ways, that's not very surprising. After all, you are well aware of the connection between your mouth and the rest of your body. You know that what goes in your mouth may eventually show up on some other part of your anatomy. You are aware of the fact that calories count; in fact, you are probably a calorie counter from way back. You may even think that "calorie" must have been one of your first words as a child!

In some ways, of course, you are right; calories *do* count. You should be more convinced than ever of their importance in the energy equation—and of the role that equation plays in weight control. Weight loss usually does involve calorie restriction. Restriction of caloric intake, however, should involve habit change, not starvation. There are important and problematical *patterns* in your calorie consumption—where, when, what, how much, and why you eat. Success lies less in counting and restricting calories than in changing the patterns involved in calorie consumption. The shift is from negative (*"don't* eat that"*) to positive ("do this to eat less"*). In the remainder of this book you'll be learning many strategies to help you eat less.

This shift to the positive may be much more important than it seems at first glance. If your emphasis is negative—"don't eat" or "eat less"—your day will be characterized by self-denial, your efforts will be expended primarily on restraint, and your focus will be on *nots.* When your resistance fails, as it will, you will wonder where your will power is when you need it!

In self-control, the emphasis is on *action,* not simply restraint. The successful self-controller focuses on eating appropriately; he assesses and modifies patterns to help him eat *and* exercise wisely. He actively practices self-control skills that lead to successful, long-term weight control.

Remember, and remember well to be a successful weight watcher, you must focus on patterns, not pounds; you must emphasize pattern change, not weight loss. Remember also that pattern change takes time. *The faster you lose weight, the more likely you are to regain it.* Quick weight loss is a sign that you are not changing long-term patterns. While your efforts may be commendable and well-intentioned, they are misplaced and unlikely to succeed unless they emphasize pattern change. Altering lifelong patterns takes more than good intentions, however. It takes concentrated effort and the development of effective skills. What are these self-control skills? How does a person learn them?

5
The Elements of
Successful Self-Control

Although research in the area of self-control was begun only recently, the evidence has already suggested some very important and practical knowledge. For example, we have already discussed the finding that self-control involves a set of complex but learnable skills. It is not an inborn and unalterable personality trait. More important, recent investigations have begun to identify and refine methods for teaching those skills. This chapter will briefly summarize the skills you will learn as you continue through the book. By way of preview, it can be stated here that *successful self-control is an exercise in personal science.* This does not mean that you need a Ph.D. in biochemistry or an interest in quantum physics. As a matter of fact, the available evidence suggests that virtually anyone can acquire effective self-control skills—regardless of his age, intelligence, or education.

What is the connection between self-control and personal science? The answer is a simple one. Judging from our current knowledge, it appears that many of the skills that help you regulate your own behavior are very similar to those used by scientists in their technical research. In self-control, of course, the science is a bit more personal since it deals with very intimate individual problems.

Both the scientist and the self-controller take an active, problem solving approach to their dilemmas. They do not resign themselves to a passive acceptance of problems or complications. Instead, they energetically question and challenge. They specify the general areas in which their problems seem to lie.

After alerting themselves to a problem and specifying its general whereabouts, both the scientist and the self-controller collect data. They attempt to improve their technical awareness by accurately observing the problem and its possible influences. This observation often involves records that allow them to review and inspect their data.

Reviewing accurate records allows them to identify important regularities or patterns. The problem may be worse at one location and better at another. It may occur predominantly on weeknights and only after 10:00 p.m. Perhaps it is often preceded by some special event (e.g., a television commercial) or followed by certain other experiences (e.g., drowsiness). These regularities frequently suggest possible sources of the problem. The late evening nibbler, for example, may conclude that his snacking is caused by food commercials or the welcome drowsiness it produces.

Identifying possible sources allows both the scientist and the self-controller to examine possible solutions. In the above example, the nibbler might consider several different options: (a) not watching television after 10:00 p.m., (b) finding alternative ways to get drowsy, (c) restricting late evening snacks to low calorie foods, (d) "saving" enough calories from supper to allow a legitimate television snack, and (e) leaving the room whenever commercials appear on the screen. The list could be much longer. In fact, the more numerous the options, the greater the likelihood that one of them will be an effective solution.

After examining his options, the individual narrows his choice to one favored candidate and then sets out to test it. This experimentation is just as important to the successful self-controller as it is to the research scientist. It is only by putting his ideas to a test that he can identify effective solutions.

The experiment, of course, requires continuing collection of evidence. The appropriateness of a given solution can be evaluated only be examining the state of the problem after the solution has been instituted. In our case of the nibbler, the individual must continue to monitor his snacking after he has begun to use his selected strategy.

Finally, the scientist and the self-controller must evaluate the adequacy of their solutions. They must examine the results of their experiment and decide on a course of action. If the test was a success, they may choose to continue and perhaps expand their use of the strategy tested. If their results were mediocre, they may want to refine or improve the strategy. And, if their experiment was a failure, they will probably want to revise their strategy or test another option.

The skills of a scientist are thus very similar to those of the successful self-controller. In both instances, the consequences of those skills are extremely rewarding. Let's review the steps in the process again with the aid of a mnemonic device. Each letter in the word SCIENCE stands for one of these valuable skills.

S *Specify* the general problem area.
C *Collect* data.
I *Identify* regularities (patterns) and possible problem sources.
E *Examine* the various options and possible solutions.
N *Narrow* the options and experiment.
C *Compare* your current data with your previous data.
E *Extend,* revise, or replace your solution.

A more detailed example might help to illustrate the critical importance of these skills in successful self-control. Let's look at the sequence from the perspective of a person who is trying to reduce.

Mrs. Smith is a happily married housewife with two young children. She has gradually acquired an extra 25 pounds over the last five years. Her concern is not only to lose some weight but also to end her pattern of picking up a few additional pounds each year.

Stage 1: Specify the general problem area. For Mrs. Smith the general problem, of course, involves an energy imbalance—she is consuming more calories than she is spending. Her goal is to identify the sources of that imbalance and to remedy it.

Stage 2: Collect data. It is hard to form an accurate picture of where things stand just by speculating about a problem. The successful reducer needs objective evidence to evaluate the nature of his or her problem. Mrs. Smith decided to use a daily diary of her eating and exercise habits. For one week, she recorded her food consumption and physical activity. This process of recording is often called "self-monitoring" or "self-observation." It is a critically important element in successful reducing. As a personal scientist, the individual needs accurate data records in order to identify regularities or patterns that may suggest the source of the problem. Mrs. Smith's diary is shown in Table 1. She chose to record food quantities rather than calories.

Stage 3: Identify patterns. After one week Mrs. Smith had a fairly accurate record of her daily food intake and activity patterns. She sat down with her diary and began looking for possible sources of her energy imbalance. On the issue of food intake, she noticed several things. First, although her meals were not terribly fattening, there was plenty of room for improvement. Her self-observation diary showed that she used mayonnaise and butter fairly regularly and that her intake of bread could be reduced without excessive suffering. She also noticed that she snacked a lot (which came as no surprise to her) and that the snacks were generally very high in calories (soda, cookies, ice cream, and so on). Snacking usually occurred midmorning, midafternoon, or late in the evening. More important, her diary allowed her to detect a potentially important exception in her snacking pattern—that she seemed less inclined to nibble when she had exercised or done something requiring moderate physical activity (see Tuesday, Thursday, and Saturday mornings; Wednesday afternoon). There were exceptions (for example, Tuesday evening), but an overall pattern was apparent.

Mrs. Smith's data records also suggested that her food quantity was not excessive. That is, even though her quality of intake could be improved, the size of her portions did not seem to be a problem. She also noticed that her coffee intake might warrant attention. As we learn in a later chapter, high caffeine intake can influence blood sugar levels and increase one's desire for sweets.

With regard to energy output, Mrs. Smith decided that her activity level was relatively low but not entirely absent. She exercised a couple of times per week and managed to include some work and play activities which required moderate amounts of calories. Thus, although she had plenty of room to increase her calorie expenditures, total inactivity did not seem to be the source of her weight problem.

Stage 4: Examine possible solutions. The source of a problem is often determined only after an effective solution has been found. In many ways, the nature of the solution tells us quite a bit about the nature of the problem. Unfortunately, it is sometimes very difficult to think of "the" solution when the source is still unknown. Personal data may suggest several different problems, each of which requires its own solution. This is one of the reasons that personal experimentation is such an important part of successful self-control.

Having reviewed her diary and suggested possible sources for her energy crisis, Mrs. Smith began to consider possible solutions. She listed changes noted on page 36.

TABLE 1

Monday, Oct. 1	Tuesday, Oct. 2	Wednesday, Oct. 3	Thursday, Oct. 4
8:30 2 pieces buttered toast, 1 bowl corn flakes with milk, 2 cups black coffee	*8:30* 1 bowl corn flakes with milk (lightly sugared), 2 cups black coffee	no breakfast (dentist appointment)	*8:45* 2 pieces buttered toast, glass of tomato juice (10 oz.), cup of coffee
10:30 4 peanut butter cookies, cup black coffee	*10:00* exercised for 30 minutes while watching Slimnastics T.V. program	*10:15* (restaurant) 2 doughnuts and cup black coffee	*10:00* exercised for 30 minutes while watching Slimnastics T.V. program
12:45 tuna fish sandwich on whole wheat toast, dill pickle, glass of milk (10 oz.), cupcake	*12:15* (restaurant) BLT sandwich, small serving coleslaw, cup of coffee	*1:00* grilled cheese sandwich with mayonnaise, 2 dill pickles, glass of V-8 juice (12 oz.)	*12:15* medium bowl vegetable soup (leftovers), half of ham sandwich, 2 cups black coffee
2:15 cup of coffee, half piece of toast with peanut butter	*3:00* 4 peanut butter cookies, 1 Coke (16 oz.)	*2:15* cleaned front closet and carried several boxes of junk to garage	*3:15* 4 graham crackers and glass of milk (12 oz.)
4:30 2 peanut butter cookies			
6:00 1 serving corn, 2 servings fish, 1 small boiled potato, 2 cups coffee	*6:00* 2 servings rice casserole, small mixed salad with dressing, 1 slice buttered bread, 1 cup coffee	*6:00* small bowl vegetable soup, 2 servings of wax beans, 1 medium chopped steak, 2 cups coffee	*6:15* 2 drumsticks and a chicken wing (Kentucky Fried), small serving coleslaw, 2 buttered rolls, 1 cup coffee
7:15 rode bicycle for 20 minutes	*7:30* walked to store (30 minutes)		
9:20 1 Coke (16 oz.) and about 25 potato chips	*9:00* 1 Dr. Pepper (16 oz.) and 6 vanilla wafers	*8:45* small bowl vanilla ice cream	

Friday, Oct. 5	Saturday, Oct. 6	Sunday, Oct. 7
8:30 bowl corn flakes with milk (no sugar),1 piece buttered toast, 2 cups coffee	*9:15* 2 slices buttered toast, 1 cup coffee	*8:45* bowl of corn flakes with milk (no sugar), 1 cup coffee
10:30 1 banana and 2 peanut butter cookies	*10:30* took kids to shopping center (probably walked 2 miles)	*11:30* 4 crackers with Cheddar cheese, 1 Pepsi (16 oz.)
11:15 softdrink (16 oz.) *12:00* ham sandwich with mayonnaise on white bread, 1 dill pickle, 6 vanilla wafers, cup of coffee	*1:00* tuna fish sandwich on whole wheat toast, 2 dill pickles, glass of milk (10 oz.)	*1:00* roast beef sandwich with mayonnaise on Roman Meal bread, 2 dill pickles, 1 buttered roll, cup of coffee
	2:45 Pepsi (16 oz.) and 2 handfuls salted peanuts	*3:30* (visited Jim's cousins) 2 cups coffee, 1 small piece fruit cake
7:00 (restaurant) 1 serving meatloaf, half scoop mashed potatoes, 1 serving mixed vegetables (peas and carrots), 2 cups coffee	*7:00* (guests for dinner) small mixed salad, 2 servings roast beef, 2 buttered rolls, 1 small baked potato with butter, 1 glass dry red wine	*6:30* (Burger Chef's) 1 fish sandwich with tartar sauce, half serving of French fries, Coke (12 oz.)
8:30 7-Up (16 oz.) and about 3 cups buttered popcorn	*8:00–11:00* 2 glasses wine, 12 crackers with Cheddar cheese, about 20 potato chips	

a. reduce calories during meals by using diet margarine, diet mayonnaise, skim milk, and other low calorie substitutes;
b. restrict daily slices of bread to a maximum of two;
c. substitute lower calorie snack items such as diet soda, unbuttered popcorn, and raw vegetables;
d. don't keep high calorie snacks in the house;
e. plan to exercise during times when snacking might occur;
f. begin drinking only decaffeinated coffee.

Stage 5: Narrow the options and experiment. After listing the above options, Mrs. Smith evaluated the likelihood of success for each one. She quickly realized that several of them would have to be modified to be reasonable. For example, it would be almost impossible to avoid having *any* high calorie snacks in the house. Her children and husband liked to snack. Similarly, it would be difficult to exercise late in the evening, when much of her snacking occurred. On the other hand, she felt that some of the remaining options were less likely to be successful. Her bread and coffee intake, for example, didn't seem that excessive.

After weighing the effort, feasibility, and probable outcome of the various options, Mrs. Smith decided to conduct a self-experiment on changing the quality of her snacking. She anticipated that this might allow her to nibble without gaining extra weight. Her experiment included a combination of two of the options she had generated. First, although she couldn't keep high calorie snacks out of the house, she began buying snacks which were her least favorite. With some welcome cooperation from her husband and children, she developed a list of snacks which they enjoyed but which did not tempt her. Sweets which were liked by both her and her family were kept out of the house. Second, she began experimenting with low calorie snacks which allowed her to nibble without getting fat. She made no-milk tapioca, unbuttered popcorn, and low calorie gelatin. Her soft drinks were replaced by diet soda, iced tea, and artificially sweetened lemonade.

Stage 6: Compare current and past data. The importance of ongoing data collection should again be emphasized. In Mrs. Smith's self-experiment, the effectiveness of her chosen option can be evaluated only by examining its results. Since permanent weight loss is often very gradual, the bathroom scale may reflect changes over long periods of time (weeks) but it is virtually worthless for day-to-day feedback on the progress of an experiment. It was therefore very important that Mrs. Smith continue her personal record keeping. Since she had focused her attention on snacking, her diary for the next two weeks included only snacking instances. Table 2 shows her data.

Mrs. Smith's evaluation of her experiment was aided by drawing a graph of her snacking. As reflected in Figure 1, her overall snacking patterns improved substantially during the two weeks of the experiment. She reduced her weekly consumption of soft drinks from eight glasses (124 ounces) in the first week to four glasses the second week and only two glasses the third. Her intake of sweets dropped from an initial level of 32 per week to nine in both of the following weeks. Peanuts, potato chips, and cheese snacks also declined.

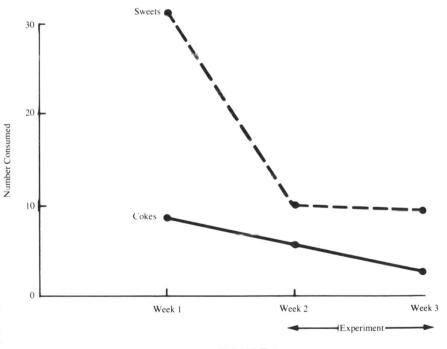

FIGURE 1

TABLE 2

Monday, Oct. 8	Tuesday, Oct. 9	Wednesday, Oct. 10	Thursday, Oct. 11
10:00 1 Diet Pepsi (16 oz.)		*10:30* small bowl of carrot & raisin salad	
	1:30 (restaurant) small piece of cake, Pepsi (16 oz.)		*2:15* Diet Pepsi (16 oz.) and four hot peppers
3:00 small bowl diet gelatin		*4:00* medium apple	
	8:15 medium bowl of carrot & raisin salad		*8:00* 3 dill pickles & glass of lemonade with saccharin (12 oz.)
8:30 3 cups unbuttered popcorn, Tab (16 oz.)		*9:00* 2 cookies (least favorite kind) and 1 Coke (16 oz.)—out of Tab	

Monday, Oct. 15	Tuesday, Oct. 16	Wednesday, Oct. 17	Thursday, Oct. 18
9:30 Fresca (16 oz.)		*10:30* bowl low calorie gelatin	*10:15* small bowl of no-milk tapioca, 1 Fresca (16 oz.)
11:30 Tab (16 oz.)			
	2:00 1 raw carrot, 2 hot peppers, 1 Diet-Rite (16 oz.)	*2:45* small apple, glass of lemonade (12 oz.) (no sugar)	*3:45* medium apple
3:15 banana			
8:15 Dr. Pepper (16 oz.)	*9:00* iced tea (12 oz.) (no sugar), 2 cookies	*8:30* 1 cupcake (Scout meeting)	*8:30* small bowl of vegetable soup

Friday, Oct. 12	Saturday, Oct. 13	Sunday, Oct. 14
10:00 Tab (16 oz.), 4 pieces raw cauliflower	*11:00* (shopping) Coke (12 oz.) and large sweet roll	*11:30* 1 doughnut, 1 Diet Pepsi (16 oz.)
3:00 glass of iced tea (16 oz.) (no sugar) and 4 pieces Melba toast	*2:30* Fresca (16 oz.) *4:30* half piece of birth-day cake	
6:00 small piece cake and 1 scoop of ice cream (Billy's birthday)	*9:00* 2 cups unbuttered popcorn, 1 7-Up (16 oz.)	*7:00* (restaurant) Coke (12 oz.) and small piece cheesecake

Friday, Oct. 19	Saturday, Oct. 20	Sunday, Oct. 21
	11:00 (shopping) 2 doughnuts, 1 soft drink (12 oz.)	*10:30* 1 glass iced tea (16 oz.) (no sugar)
2:00 2 pieces Halloween candy, 1 Fresca (16 oz.)	*3:15* small bowl of low calorie gelatin	*2:15* 4 hot peppers, 1 dill pickle *4:00* cupcake
8:00 2 cups unbuttered popcorn, 1 Diet Rite (16 oz.)	*7:30–11:00* (guests) 2 small pieces cake, 1 Tab (16 oz.)	*8:30* small tossed salad

Relative to her previous snacking behavior, then, Mrs. Smith's nibbling had dramatically improved. Notice that she did not *eliminate* sweets—she just cut back on them. The importance of avoiding perfectionistic goals will be emphasized in the next chapter. For the time being, it should be noted that Mrs. Smith allowed herself flexibility in her self-control efforts. Also note that her continuing data diary not only provided information on the results of her experiment but also offered additional information for generating revised problem solutions. For example, from her two-week experimental records she noticed that many of her snacking problems occurred on weekends. This suggested further options for improving her snacking patterns.

Stage 7: Extend, revise, or replace your solution. Mrs. Smith decided that her chosen self-control strategy had worked fairly well. With the exception of some occasional high calorie snacks, she had developed some adaptive nibbling patterns which allowed her to snack without consuming excessive calories. Although she didn't want to eliminate sweets totally, she decided to attempt some further improvement in weekend snacking. In addition to continuing her experimental strategy, she began preparing low calorie snacks on Saturday morning to provide her with legitimate options for weekend snacks.

The above illustration is only one of many which will be offered in this book. As you progress from one chapter to the next, the personal science sequence will become a familiar and beneficial guideline in your own successful reducing. Before previewing the remaining chapters, however, a review and discussion of that critically important sequence may be worthwhile.

Stage 1: Specify the general problem area. In reducing, the most obvious problem is an energy imbalance. But is it food *quality* (high calorie foods) or food *quantity* (extra large portions)? To what extent is physical inactivity a factor? If the problem stems from snacking, what are the factors that surround snacking? Can a large percent of your excess calories be traced to a couple of habits or problem foods (cheese, sweets, wine, soda, etc.)?

Stage 2: Collect data. The crucial role of *accurate* personal records cannot be overemphasized. Many a weight watcher has been amazed to find that his self-monitored eating habits were very different from what he would have guessed. General estimates and self-evaluations based on "retrospective data" are notoriously inaccurate in self-control. Research studies have shown that dieters' estimates of their caloric intake are often grossly inaccurate. The moral here is that you cannot rely on guessing or memory to discover the source of a problematical pattern. Even though they are sometimes cumbersome and boring, accurate self-records are an indispensable aspect of successful self-control. As your skills in personal science improve, the need for continuous self-monitoring will probably decrease. However, in attacking new problems or wrestling with complications in old ones, personal data reign supreme. As one researcher has put it, the successful self-controller must "care enough to count."

There are, of course, many different ways to collect data and an infinite number of potential targets. One can count calories, grams, ounces, or servings. The target might be sweets, soda, dietetic foods, or virtually any category of intake. For energy expenditure, personal records may tally specific exercises or duration of an activity.

The cardinal rule in personal data collection is this: *adopt the record keeping system that offers the best balance of accuracy, relevance, and ease.* In other words, make your counting count. If a recording system is inaccurate because of its vagueness or its difficulty, it will be of little use in your reduction efforts. *Effective personal science requires accurate personal data.* But the data must also be relevant. Counting consumption of sweets will help little if your primary problems do not stem from excessive sweets. Moreover, there may be many other aspects of your everyday life that merit recording. A daily tally of candy consumption gives you a summary figure on the frequency of this behavior, but it may tell you very little about some of the patterns in your candy capers. For example, are they associated with times of the day? days of the week? physical locations? certain previous thoughts or events? Later chapters in this book will illustrate some personal record keeping systems that collect data on the frequency of a behavior, its physical location, the time of day, and any associated events. These systems can be invaluable in reflecting patterns and suggesting possible problem sources.

An accurate and relevant data system is useful, however, only if it is feasible. Systems that require a lot of work may encourage dishonesty and will seldom last more than a few days. Counting calories or bites, for example, is a very difficult enterprise for most reducers. More reasonable systems provide useful data without imposing excessive demands on the individual.

Stage 3: Identify patterns. Does the problem behavior occur at regular times (afternoons, weekends, etc.)? Is it associated with a particular place, person, thought, or activity? Are there notable exceptions when the behavior does not occur? What usually precedes it? What follows it?

These are the kinds of questions that can be asked in examining personal data for patterns and potential problem sources. It is important in this stage to consider many possible sources.

Stage 4: Examine possible solutions. What are the various ways of changing a problematical pattern? Can you rearrange your physical environment to reduce the behavior? How about your social environment? Are there elements in your "private environment"—the things you say to yourself, your standards, and so on—that might be altered? Can you substitute or increase an alternative behavior?

At this stage of personal science, the generation of many different options is desirable. Try to think of innovative or bizarre solutions—they may turn out to be the best. In addition, when you think of a possible solution, try to fantasize your pursuit of it. Generate a mental movie in which you see yourself going through the actions required by the solution. This mental rehearsal will often help you to anticipate possible complications and make improvements in your self-control strategy.

Stage 5: Narrow the options and experiment. Evaluate your options critically. Begin by eliminating those that seem unfeasible. Next, drop those that are least likely to change your problem behavior. From the remaining, combine promising elements or choose the option that seems most likely to succeed. Your choice should evaluate feasibility, effort, and probable success. Don't pick a solution that requires Herculean effort or excessive attention.

Stage 6: Compare current and past data. Beware of perfectionism here. Your problem behavior doesn't have to be totally eliminated for your experiment to be a success. Has the pattern changed at all? Do you have enough data to decide? Would another week of experimentation help determine effectiveness?

A graph or chart is often helpful in this stage. Also, beware of hasty conclusions. If your experiment lasted less than two weeks, it is probably too early to conclude anything from your data. You should also watch for confounding circumstances—factors other than your chosen strategy that may have influenced the problem behavior.

Stage 7: Extend, revise, or replace your solution. If the selected strategy was mildly or moderately successful, how could it be improved? can it be streamlined or refined before continuation? If the strategy failed, consider the possible reasons. Are your data really accurate? Did you use the strategy consistently? Was your experiment too brief? Were there other factors working against success? Was your strategy too ambitious or not ambitious enough? Which of the other options might have been a better choice?

We often learn more from one mistake than from ten correct solutions. Learning to accept our capacity to make mistakes is itself a valuable lesson. Personal science thrives on trial and error learning, and the "error" component is an important one. Be prepared to "hang in there" with a revision and another try. When you learn from your mistakes, failure is an impossibility. You will undoubtedly lose a few battles in winning a very important war.

The remainder of this book provides additional applications of the personal science program in a variety of weight control areas. You will learn how to assess and resolve problems in nutrition, motivation, and activity patterns. Technical suggestions will be offered on how to develop a supportive social environment. You will learn to assess and, if necessary, modify various aspects of your energy crisis—your eating style, cues that influence hunger, and nervous eating. Most important, you will develop independent skills as a personal scientist which will allow you to extend and improve your self-control.

Weight control researchers often talk about this or that technique as if it were a *universal* solution to obesity. Their experiments are often aimed at identifying these universals. However, the most relevant weight control data for you are not found in technical journals. The most relevant data for you are your own. Universal solutions to obesity are probably nonexistent. Each person is a unique and complex combination of factors which influence energy balance. Successful self-control strategies must therefore be personalized to meet the needs of the individual. In personal science, suggestions are drawn from formal research, but the critical data are your own. Regardless of popular opinion and formal scientific consensus, if a strategy works for *you* it should be adopted. The personal scientist is committed to self-improvement through a systematic self-corrective sequence.

You may have noticed that we have not yet mentioned weight loss goals or poundage charts. For most dieters, the real test of their progress is the scale. There, in the cold light of dawn, they anxiously place their feet on a little platform that can bring either depression or delight. Like a somber roulette wheel, the numbers roll past a little window. Where they stop often determines the dieter's state of mind for the next 24 hours.

If your day-to-day motivation fluctuates with the feedback you receive from your bathroom scale, then *frequent weigh-ins may be a destructive element in your reducing program*. The average home scale is not accurate enough to detect weight changes of one to two pounds. Moreover, daily fluctuations in weight often reflect differences in fluid retention or foot placement. Most people do not lose a pound of *fat* overnight. As a matter of fact, if you are losing much more than one percent of your bodyweight per week, it is likely that you are *not* losing just fat. Body fluids and "lean body mass" (muscles and certain organs) are frequently sacrificed in crash reduction programs.

A second side effect of frequent weigh-ins is the undue emphasis they place on pounds. You are now aware that *people who emphasize "weight loss" over "habit change" are often less successful in their long-term reduction*. Emphasizing pounds may distract your efforts from the real culprits in obesity—the behavior patterns that make up your eating and activity habits. Ultimate weight loss, of course, is the goal of any reducing program, but it is most successfully attained by focusing on altering personal patterns relevant to energy balance by the persistent application of self-control skills. The moral here—and it cannot be overemphasized—is THINK BEHAVIOR.

Occasional weigh-ins will help to give you a quantified assurance of progress without allowing the scale to dominate your life. We recommend that you *weigh yourself no more often then every two weeks*. If you are a veteran dieter, it will be hard to stay away from the scale during the first part of the program. Your curiosity will beg for a weigh-in, if just to see whether a miracle is in the making. Be prepared—there is no miracle. Permanent weight loss is a difficult and slow undertaking. The extra pounds you have acquired stem from eating and activity patterns that have become comfortable parts of your lifestyle. They have been around for years and are probably a bit set in their ways. Enduring self-control is an exercise in active patience. You must work actively to improve both your skills and your energy patterns. At the same time you must be patient and reasonable in pacing your self-renovation. Don't expect a "new you" in six weeks unless the "old you" was equally rapid in creation.

Our caution here should *not* be taken lightly. Successful self-control is an immensely valuable and rewarding endeavor. However, we would be dishonest to claim that it is easy, simple, or quickly attained. It is typically none of these. It involves skills you can learn and requires efforts that are equal to their outcomes. Its progress is measured in weeks and months rather than days, but its rewarding consequences are often witnessed for many years.

To receive maximum benefits from this book, it should be read chapter by chapter in the sequence presented. Becoming an effective personal scientist requires the pursuit of information in an organized, step-by-step fashion. All too often, the overly enthusiastic self-controller aborts his own attempt before it gets off the ground by undertaking too much, too quickly. Just as a scientific approach is a step-by-step procedure, so must be the development of skills in utilizing that approach. However, some of you may find it difficult to curb your curiosity about later chapters. If so, we recommend that you scan the book briefly, and then begin your personal science program. At that time, it is critically important that your efforts be focused individually on each chapter and its assignment in the sequence presented. Be sure to devote the recommended amount of time and effort to each part of an assignment before continuing.

We also recommend that you adopt an additive or cumulative strategy as your skills develop. Each topic of focus will request several weeks of your time. As you move on to the next unit, do not simply throw the old one out the window—build on it. Move on to each new assignment only when the previous one is running fairly smoothly and, as much as possible, continue any previously successful experiments as you expand to new ones. This will help you to maintain previous progress as you make further inroads into your weight problem. As you develop comfortably thinner patterns of eating and activity, it will become progressively easier to shift your primary attention to a new topic and a new assignment. We recommend that you occasionally review previous chapters to assist you in this process.

6
Cognitive Ecology: Cleaning Up What You Say to Yourself

Having learned that a successful self-controller is a practicing personal scientist, you are now ready to apply your skills in an area that lies at the core of self-change. You are ready for the inside story of most self-control successes.

How many times have you heard, perhaps quoted, some variation of the old adage, "You are what you think"? To many of us, it strikes a familiar note. You may not realize, however, that the idea it captures may well be the most significant factor in the success or failure of your personal self-change efforts. That idea can be summarized very simply: *what you say to yourself makes a difference.* It may make *the* difference in whether six months (or ten years) from now you will be defeated or delighted as your own personal scientist. Your inside story may even make the difference in whether you are alive, and healthy enough, to enjoy telling it.

Now, you may be saying to yourself, those are rather dramatic statements to make, aren't they? If so, you have already taken an important first step in assuming the attitude of a scientist: an evaluative, critical attitude about any new information you encounter. Let's check it out.

You, like most human beings, *think a lot.* Most of your life is spent in the privacy of your own head. Your waking hours are enacted in an unending sequence of thoughts, reveries, daydreams, memories, and plans. Even when you are sleeping your head is not idle, as anyone who has awakened with a start from a bad dream can attest. Your *cognitions* (which may be thoughts or images—mental pictures) are your constant companions. In some ways they are your most valuable companions; your ability to think sets you apart from the rest of our world in several important ways. Cognitions allow you to remember and to use your past experiences in your current decisions and behaviors. They also allow you to anticipate the results of various decisions and solutions without actually having to *enact* each of them. It is fascinating to realize that your cognitive abilities allow you to *imagine* places you've never been, things you've never done, people you've never met. However, perhaps the most impressive skill your brain gives to you is the ability to figure out problems you've never solved before. By utilizing your memories of past experiences, your anticipation of future consequences, and your awareness of your present situation, you can become an effective problem solver in the here-and-now. And, as you've already learned, that's what self-control and personal science are all about.

Your cognitions are important in and of themselves. Further, they exert an important influence on your behavior and your emotions. Regardless of your sex, age, or physiology, *your thoughts and images strongly affect the way you behave and the way you feel*. No one is immune to the effects of his own cognitive environment. This point has been demonstrated repeatedly by scientific research with various groups and various problems. It has been shown that individuals' thoughts affect their ability to tolerate pain. Impulsive children, who find it difficult to concentrate on and complete a task, are greatly affected by what they are saying to themselves. Self-talk has also been shown to be a major component in the extreme fears of some people, fears which prohibit or limit their activities. Most important for you, your cognitions may be a critical factor in your own eating patterns. Eating is often a response to internal cues: thoughts and feelings.

Let's bring that point a little closer to home. How many times per day do you think about or imagine that box of cookies in the cabinet, that casserole you're going to make for dinner, that luscious piece of cake you ate for lunch? Makes your mouth water just to think about it, doesn't it? It certainly does! And how many times per day do those thoughts and images cue you to go to the kitchen for another sliver of cake or just a couple of cookies?

Now, what happens next? You've finished your sliver of cake (which turned out to be three or four). You've gone back to your book and are attempting to get back into that good chapter you're trying to finish before the kids get home from school. But your head keeps returning to that scene in the kitchen. And sure enough, this time your thoughts are on the other side of the fence: "Well, you just blew it, didn't you? You weren't even hungry and you stuffed yourself anyway. You deserve to be fat!" One thought leads to another, and very soon you start to *feel* bad—frustrated, disgusted, angry at yourself. Within minutes you've talked yourself into *feeling* depressed and defeated. "I'll never make it anyway; I might as well give up. It's just too much effort; apparently I don't have what it takes." Those relentless thoughts are at it again—and pretty soon you're back in the kitchen!

Familiar—and frustrating, isn't it? The very familiarity of this cycle may have prevented you from standing back and looking at the role your thoughts play in initiating and maintaining that vicious cycle. You may well be asking yourself at this point, "If my ability to think is such a great thing to have, why do I get stuck in these miserable cycles?" That's a good question—and, fortunately, one for which there's a good answer. Careful examination suggests that it's not your *ability* to think or talk to yourself that gets you into trouble; it's *what* you talk to yourself *about*. *What* you say to yourself makes the critical difference in how you feel and how you act.

You can learn to control what you think about. You can get that cycle to work for you instead of against you by cleaning up and rearranging your cognitive environment. That cycle can become your best friend instead of your worst enemy. Why have we emphasized the negative aspects so strongly? If you have a weight problem (an "eating" problem), it's a fairly safe bet that your cognitive ecology needs improvement. You may be a compulsively neat, meticulous person—and still be a cognitive garbage collector whose thoughts are cluttered with self-criticisms and unrealistic standards, polluted with negative predictions and self-defeating monologues. The most important part of your anatomy for successful weight control is your *head,* not your stomach. Your brain is your *most* vital organ.

Fortunately, you *can* clean up your cognitions; you can change the content of your thoughts and images, which in turn can influence your behaviors and your feelings. The rest of this chapter will be devoted to teaching you how to specify your frequent maladaptive cognitions and how to replace them with appropriate, helpful ones.

Let's stop for a moment and be sure you are thinking clearly right now. We have suggested three important ideas: 1) you, as a human being, think a lot; 2) the content of your thoughts (and images) influences your behavior and your feelings; and 3) you can learn to control the content of your thoughts by changing what you think *about* or say to yourself. Your first experience as a personal scientist may well be in the area most important to your long-term success. We hope this clarification of the role of your thoughts in self-change has helped to dispel any lingering attachment on your part to the notion of will power. It should be clear that the individuals to whom you have attributed brute strength when it comes to self-control are actually skilled cognitive custodians. They have learned to talk to themselves in optimistic but realistic ways. Further, they are people who realize that cognitive housecleaning is a time-consuming endeavor. Appropriate self-talk *typically* takes months, even years, to develop; it is a prime example of our principle: effort equals outcome. Self-controllers also know that there is frequently a lag between changed self-talk and changed feelings; that is, it takes time for new thoughts to help produce new feelings. If you are not prepared for that lag, you may easily become discouraged.

This cautionary word should suggest to you that there are some vital differences in this problem-solving approach to cognitive ecology and the "power of positive thinking" approaches familiar to most of us. Some important discrepancies can be delineated. Let's label our approach of changing what you say to yourself as cognitive restructuring. It emphasizes realistic, behavior-oriented self-statements as opposed to the unrealistic "autosuggestions" offered by many best sellers. Cognitive restructuring places simultaneous emphasis on performance tasks related to your new, relevant self-statements. In other words, it teaches you to practice what you preach, after first making sure your sermon topics are realistic. This is in sharp contrast to Madison Avenue "miracles" supposedly wrought by thought control systems. Finally, what follows is based on data collected in clinical laboratories by scientists using the same approach you will be applying. It has been demonstrated that those impulsive children, those fearful adults (and institutionalized individuals, elderly people, and many others) can change their behaviors and their feelings by talking to themselves differently.

Good cognitive ecology is a difficult, time-consuming pursuit, but one that promises you literal "lifetime returns." It begins with an understanding of your current cognitive contents.

As you tackle your cognitive housecleaning, what are the problem spots you're most likely to encounter? Two categories of thoughts that subtly sabotage many self-change attempts are *personal goals* and *private monologues*. Your personal "junk box" may be replete with other problem thoughts that are more frequent saboteurs of your efforts to improve your eating patterns. These two categories, however, are your most probable culprits; they can aptly serve as examples of other problematical cognitions.

PERSONAL GOALS

The first step in your cognitive housecleaning is to learn to set reasonable goals. Now, that sounds easy enough, doesn't it? You are, in all likelihood, an accomplished goal setter; you probably learned a long time ago that you accomplish more—in less time—when you decide in advance just what you want to accomplish and how you're going to go about it. You may have even noted that goal setting is especially important in the area of self-change. In general, it is easier to modify a problem behavior if you specify precisely what you want to change it *to*.

If goals are so important to self-change, and if you've had so much practice setting them, then what's the problem? The problem lies, not in the act of setting goals, but in the kinds of goals many people set. Before we examine some of those inappropriate goals, let's first take a more careful look at what a goal actually involves. *What are the parts or ingredients of a goal?*

A goal has at least two parts: an *active* and a *reactive* ingredient. The active ingredient is the familiar one we've already discussed: a goal typically specifies something you're going to *do*. You may want to maintain, initiate, increase, decrease, or eliminate some behavior or thought. Each of these alternatives implies an *action* on your part.

The second ingredient, the *reactive* one, may not sound quite so familiar. Each goal you set has one of three possible outcomes: you may achieve it, exceed it, or fall short of it. Each of these outcomes elicits some *reaction* from you. If you achieve it or exceed it, you may give yourself a pat on the back; if you fall short of it, you may give yourself a nudge to do better next time. Each of these reactions affects the way you feel about yourself.

Your personal goals, then, exert considerable influence on both your behavior and your feelings; they specify an action and involve a reaction. Now that you have a better grasp of the meaning and the importance of your goals, let's see where they may be getting you into trouble.

The Pitfall of Perfectionism

You may be the fortunate individual who has already learned to set moderate, reasonable goals, or you may be the less fortunate person who has learned to set goals that are too simple to provide any challenge. In our achievement-oriented culture, however, you are probably the unfortunate person who has learned to set goals that are rigid and perfectionistic. If so, you may be an expert in engineering your own self-defeat. Perfectionism is the number one enemy of problem solving.

What kind of goals do you usually set? Are they frequently "never" or "always" statements? Are they often a reflection of all-or-none perfectionistic thinking? How frequently do you decide that you will *never* eat another doughnut, or that you will *always* drink your coffee black? If your goals are unreasonable and inflexible, you are setting yourself up for problems, not solutions, in your self-control efforts.

"O.K.," you may be thinking, "so my goals are a little bit high. What's so bad about that?" Let's find out, keeping in mind the effect of your goals on your behavior and your emotions. First, all-or-nothing goals encourage all-or-nothing behavior. A "never" or "always" goal defines your success precisely in those terms; to succeed you must *never* eat a dessert again. You are asking yourself for perfect behavior, for errorless eating habits. You are leaving yourself no room for human error, for *gradual* improvement. You are constantly living *one* mistake away from failure, one error away from defeat. One violation—and you've blown it; you're "off your diet." In your own self-defined terms, you're either a saint or a sinner, a complete success or a total failure.

Now, what is the probability, especially in terms of your past consumer history, that you will never eat a dessert again? If you are as human as most people are, it is very, very low; human beings are notoriously bad at being perfect! Suppose it's Monday morning. After a weekend of indulgence (Aunt May brought over a pan of brownies, which she *knows* are your weakness, on Saturday), you've decided to eliminate brownies from your diet—*permanently!* No more fooling around with half-hearted attempts at dieting! What a good feeling to set a goal for yourself, and to anticipate a new, slimmer you! Monday's not such a bad day after all (especially since you still feel full from your weekend eating). All day Monday and Tuesday you give yourself frequent reminders of your new goal, just to keep temptation from rearing its ugly, familiar head. Then, late on Tuesday, an interesting thing happens; those brownies, so easily given up yesterday, start to sound a little better. But you stand firm. You've set a goal and you're going to reach it. After all, it's not like you've given up *food*—just one kind. Surely, that's not so hard. Anybody can do that. It just takes will power—and this time you're going to show yourself you've got it!

Wednesday rolls around, and you spend most of the day rehearsing all the reasons that brownies are bad for you; at bedtime you notice that brownies seem to have dominated your day. But at least you didn't eat one even though Aunt May, noting how much you enjoyed them, brought over another half dozen—which you fed to the kids. By Thursday you notice that all the reminders you give yourself are starting to elicit a different reaction. Every time you think about brownies—and those thoughts seem to be increasing in frequency—you feel angry and cheated. It's not *fair* that you should have to give up something you enjoy so much! Why should *you* have to give them up when the kids—and everyone else you know—can eat all they want? You feel increasingly resentful, dominated, and suffocated by your own self-deprivation.

This phenomenon, called "cognitive claustrophobia," is a very frequent occurrence. Goals that are too rigid often generate a list of forbidden fruits; ironically, prohibition is a very good way to increase the temptation value of a food (as well as other items). The more rigidly you deprive yourself of a particular food, the more you seem to want it. You find yourself obsessed with a brownie, a difficulty which your skinny friends may have trouble appreciating but which causes you a great deal of frustration and resentment.

The active and reactive ingredients of a goal become very apparent here; let's get back to you and that brownie and see how they interact. Where are we most likely to find you after a couple of days of self-denial and a great deal of resentment? Many of you can guess. In all likelihood you are at the bakery, buying, not one or two, but a *dozen* brownies—and maybe a couple of cupcakes to boot.

Cognitive claustrophobia, a feeling that results from perfectionistic thinking, leads to binge eating, the very behavior you'd most like to avoid. If *one* brownie is going to blow it—and with your goal, it is—then you might as well eat a dozen. Your goal has affected your behavior—adversely. What further influence does it have on your emotions? You may well feel an initial sense of relief when you start a binge—and understandably so: once you have erred, you are temporarily freed from your rigid goal for that day. At the end of your binge, however, you are very likely to feel depressed, guilty, and self-critical. This is a vicious cycle, indeed—one that takes its toll on your eating patterns *and* your feelings about yourself. If you've experienced it, you are well aware of its negative consequences; it is an exercise in self-defeat.

Now, let's stop and tie things together. You have seen that your goals are important—possibly more important than you have realized. Their importance lies in their effects on your eating *behavior* and your eating emotions. Ironically, goals can be one of your greatest hindrances. It is easy to see why they deserve consideration in your personal cognitive cleanup. If goals can create such a problematical cycle—if they can leave you further back than where you started—why set them? Why would a personal scientist insist that goals are an essential part of an effective problem-solving sequence?

The problem lies, not in goal setting itself, but in the *kinds* of goals that are set. Part of becoming an efficient personal scientist—and the first step in cleaning up your cognitive ecology—is to learn to set *reasonable* goals. It will soon be apparent that goals can be a help as well as a hindrance.

What Are Some Guidelines for Setting Goals?

Appropriate goal setting, like self-control, is a learnable skill; it involves careful adherence to a few general guidelines. A personal scientist sets goals that are specific, reasonable, and flexible.

Set specific behavior goals. "I will *be*" goals should be replaced with "I will *do*" goals. Many people establish goals of improving personal traits or characteristics, such as "developing will power." There is little evidence that individuals possess general traits; even if they did, setting goals in those terms would be a misguided attempt. Goals should tell you precisely *what* you are trying to achieve; otherwise you will never know if you've achieved it! Like will power, most traits are measurable only in behavioral terms. You attribute will power and other traits to others on the basis of their *behaviors*.

Effective goals provide a guideline for action. They specify precisely what you are going to change, tell you specifically how you are going to behave. In so doing, they provide a precise, accurate measure of your success or failure in achieving your goal.

Let's look at another common mistake. Goals may be specific and still fail to specify a *behavior*. A prime example is the frequent setting of "pounds" goals. Let's say you've resolved to lose 20 pounds. That's specific, isn't it? Specific numerically? Yes. Specific behaviorally? No. You cannot directly change that number on your scale; you can only change behaviors that result in a lower number on your scale.

The only route to pounds lost or to any other goal is changed behavior. *Set your goals in behavior terms*—and the pounds and the traits will take care of themselves. Remember—think BEHAVIOR.

Set reasonable goals. You've already learned about the disastrous consequences of setting unreasonable, perfectionistic goals. We hope you've decided that your future goals are going to be realistic and reasonable, as well as behaviorally specific. Your next question may well be, "How can I tell if my goals are reasonable?" If so, you're thinking straight. It's one thing to resolve to set realistic goals; it's quite another thing to know *how* to do it.

What is a reasonable goal? *A reasonable goal is,* first and foremost, *a relative goal.* A reasonable goal is relative—and relative to one criterion only. That criterion is your own past and current behavior. Realistic goals reflect where you have been, as well as where you are going. This is one instance in which hindsight may well be better than foresight.

Your goals must be specific to you; self-control efforts start where you are *now*. If your goal is to increase the amount of exercise you get on a daily basis, your first question should be, "How much exercise do I *usually* get per day?" Here's where data collection comes in handy. An accurate picture of your current behavior is essential to effective goal-setting. If you find that your daily exercise consists of two or three trips up and down your basement steps, it would be unrealistic and self-defeating to plan to do 50 sit-ups per day. If you are already doing 40 per day, however, it might be quite reasonable to add another ten. Let's take another example. If you are snacking five or six times per day, it might be reasonable initially to cut down to three or four. It probably would not be reasonable to eliminate all but one.

These are specific examples of a general principle whose importance cannot be overemphasized. Your current behavior—and *only* your current behavior—should serve as *your* goal-setting guideline. If your friend Jane can eat five snacks a day and still lose weight, good for her. If your husband exercises five times a week—and loves it— good for him. If your children are bottomless pits—and beanpoles— good for them. No one but you has your unique combination of metabolism, physiology, and past behavioral (eating) history. No goal is reasonable in and of itself; it can only be reasonable *for you*. The golden rule of goal setting is that reasonable goals are relative goals.

Now, let's say you've pinpointed a problem area, you've collected data on your current behavior, and you're ready to set a goal. You have found, to your surprise, that coffee breaks at work are your downfall. Those occasional morning sweetrolls and afternoon candy bars have gotten to be the rule, not the exception. In fact, your data from last week showed only one coffee break out of ten that was actually a *coffee break*. And that was the day you had eaten cheesecake for lunch. You've figured out that a high percentage of your weekly junk calories have been those snacks you're gulping down to tide you over until lunch or dinner.

You've specified a problem; you have a clear picture of your current behavior. You know that a reasonable goal specifies a behavior that is a *small* step away from your current behavior. But you're still not sure what's reasonable; how small should each step be? Should you cut back on your daily snacks by 50 percent per week, 30 percent, 10 percent, until you're down to one or two snacks per week? You're eager to change that pattern as quickly as possible; you don't want to waste time by setting goals that are too easy to attain. Yet you certainly don't want to program failure by setting goals that are unreasonable.

How do you know, ahead of time, what goals will be easy enough to achieve, but difficult enough to challenge? You can't know—for certain. You may set a goal that *seems* reasonable relative to your current behavior—and find that it represented too big a step. Or vice versa. You can't know for sure how easy a goal will be until you try it.

There are, however, at least two strategies that will help you make a best guess.

The first of these involves making a mental movie, in which you are the producer, director, star—and critic. Mental movies, you may remember, can be very helpful in the generation of appropriate solutions in the problem solving sequence. One useful way to evaluate the reasonableness of a goal is to *picture* yourself performing the new behavior it specifies. Let's get back to your coffee breaks. You've decided to eliminate your afternoon snack, reduction of approximately 50 percent per week. That seems a little high in terms of your current behavior—but there's no logical reason it should be. After all, by break time in the afternoon you've already had two meals and a snack, and it's only three hours until dinner. Just to be on the safe side, you decide to check it out with a mental rehearsal. You picture yourself, as clearly as possible, walking over to the corner drugstore with your coworkers. You listen in on the usual conversation; you hear more about Al's fantastic weekend, Mary's dinner plans, and Diane's new promotion. With your "other ear" you listen to your own self-talk; you can hear your self-instructions about ordering coffee—and only coffee. Next, you picture yourself sitting in your favorite booth, listening to the orders of your friends. Now, you really try to zero in on your own thoughts and feelings. You concentrate on imagining your thoughts and feelings as you drink your coffee, watching your coworkers downing their milkshakes and sundaes. How do you feel? What are you thinking about?

You may be surprised to find out that mental rehearsal can project you into a situation with surprising vividness. You may be even more surprised to find that visualizing yourself in a situation may elicit thoughts and feelings you are likely to encounter in the actual situation. You are the star performer in your mental movies; you are also your major critic. Imagining yourself in problem situations may give you an opportunity to modify your goals without actually having to try them out. For example, as you see yourself sipping coffee, minus your usual candy bar, you might notice that you are making constant comparisons between your coffee and your friends' desserts. Cues such as this may influence you to modify your goal to the substitution of a low calorie snack at afternoon coffee break.

Mental rehearsal is a valuable strategy in the testing of a goal; it can also be a useful technique to use in practicing a new behavior. When you feel relatively confident that a behavioral goal *is* reasonable, you can imagine yourself performing it several times before the situation actually occurs. The more prepared you are for the actual situation, the more likely you are to perform the desirable behavior in that situation.

The second strategy for evaluating the reasonableness of your goal involves your playing therapist. Let's pretend that your best friend has just come to you for some much needed assistance and support. Now, let's assign to her the exact problem you are facing and the tentative goal you have set. What would you say to her? If your problem were her problem, would you set the same goal? A very provocative question in the evaluation of your goals could be: would I set this goal for another person who has my problem and my personal history? If not, perhaps your goal deserves reconsideration.

Your chances of setting appropriate goals are greatly improved by using your current behavior as your guideline; they are increased even further by testing the goal through a mental rehearsal or through its imagined imposition on another person. You must remember, however, that a personal scientist deals in best guesses, not final answers. Personal science progresses through a thoughtful trial and error process. The efficient self-controller constantly remains open to changing circumstances and alternative solutions.

Set flexible goals. In the final analysis, you cannot know whether a goal is reasonable or unreasonable until you have attempted to achieve it. Repeated failure at performing the new behavior specified by your goal should raise the question of whether the step from your current to the new behavior is too large. Don't misunderstand; a reasonable goal is not a goal that poses no challenge. You should expect some difficulty in performing *new* behaviors in *old* familiar situations. You will learn more in later chapters about ways to program that new behavior ahead of time. But repeated failure, despite your practice through mental rehearsal and encouraging self-talk, means that your goal may be unrealistic. Back up a step or two, and try again. If your goals are not helpful, there is something wrong with them, not with you.

If you have decided to set and to evaluate your goals in terms of these guidelines, you are well on your way to an improved cognitive ecology. Let's take a brief look at another frequent cognitive culprit that may be sabotaging your self-change efforts—your private monologues.

PRIVATE MONOLOGUES

Suppose you are in the supermarket, deliberating over what variety of diet soda you are going to buy this week. Suddenly you hear a loud, familiar voice that tells you your least favorite aunt is in the vicinity. "What are you buying that low calorie stuff for? You know everybody in our family is chubby!" Good old Aunt Clara. Some relatives you could do without, right? That kind of statement is the last thing you need in your weight control efforts; it is discouraging and depressing. You feel legitimately angry and disgusted with Aunt Clara and her unwanted remarks.

Yet—how many times do *you* talk to yourself in discouraging, self-defeating ways? You may be guilty of more negative, inappropriate self-talk in a week than you hear from others in a month or more. No one else would have the nerve to say to you some of the things you say to yourself!

The *second step in improving your cognitive ecology is to replace your negative monologues with more appropriate ones.* You spend a lifetime talking to yourself; you've already learned that your conversations with yourself have a powerful impact on your behavior and your feelings. If your past self-control efforts have gone the way of many good intentions, your private monologues may be the culprit. Let's look at some typical examples of self-defeating self-talk, and then see what you can do to change them.

Negative or maladaptive monologues frequently occur as the reactive ingredient of a perfectionistic goal. Let's review for a moment. We have seen how people frequently react to perfectionistic goal setting with feelings of resentment and depression. What are some of the things you're likely to be saying to yourself when this phenomenon occurs? In the first part of the cycle, when you're rigidly adhering to that goal you've set, you're likely to be engaged in a private monologue such as:

> It's just *not* fair. Here I am, starving myself, and so far (after three days) I haven't lost a single pound. All my friends can eat all they want; everything I eat turns right to fat. I've given up my favorite foods—and what have I gotten for it? Nothing. And I probably won't. I never lose anything, no matter how hard I try.

How long would it take for this kind of self-talk to result in feelings of anger and frustration—and eventually in the binges that often follow rigid self-deprivation? Probably not long. On the basis of three days of effort, this misguided self-controller has concluded he is the most unfortunate person he knows, and that he will never lose weight, regardless of his efforts. He has turned a frustrating situation into a catastrophe. Catastrophizing—exaggerating the negative aspects of a situation—frequently gets in the way of effective problem solving. It is a frequent characteristic of negative monologues.

Next, suppose this self-defeating fellow has talked himself into a binge, an initially welcome release from his self-imposed deprivation. Relief is soon replaced by depression and guilt. Now, what's he saying to himself? His self-talk probably sounds something like this:

> Well, I blew it. I did it again. What is wrong with me? I never do anything right. Everything I try ends up the same way. Nothing I do works. I'm just a failure. Whatever it takes, I don't have it. I'm always going to be a fat slob.

It is not too hard to see why feelings of depression and worthlessness accompany binge eating. This kind of self-talk virtually guarantees self-defeat. Notice the emphasis on general trait statements, such as "I *am* a failure" and "I'm always going to *be* a fat slob." The implication is a deep-seated personal inadequacy rather than a behavioral deficiency. Talking to yourself about traits is both unjustified and self-defeating; traits are not amenable to change. Behaviors are. We are not suggesting here that all behavior deserves glowing praise, or even approval. We are suggesting, however, that your self-talk can be realistic without being punitive or pessimistic.

Maladaptive monologues are not limited to reactions to rigid, unrealistic goals; they occur on many occasions about many topics. Individuals may repeatedly sabotage their own efforts by focusing their self-talk on traits, pounds, excuses, food—the list is endless. Only the outcome is the same; inappropirate self-talk contributes to inappropriate behavior. Negative self-talk leads to negative feelings—feelings of anger, frustration, guilt, and depression.

People who have a high frequency of negative self-talk also, not surprisingly, have a low frequency of positive self-talk. The rule of thumb for many individuals seems to be: if you can't say something *bad* about yourself, don't say anything at all! It is sad, but true, that our culture often frowns upon positive self-evaluation, even when it's justified. Observe the response you get the next time you pay someone a genuine, well-deserved compliment. If the person says ''Thank you,'' he's an exception. He, or she, is more likely to play down the good job he did by saying something like: ''Well, you know I had a lot of help'' or ''Anyone could have done it.'' It seems that the individuals who are most likely to be self-critical are the most unlikely to be self-praising. If you praised your spouse or your children with the same frequency with which you praise yourself, would they continue to behave in ways you like? How do you feel when you do a good job at something and get no positive feedback? Yet you—who are more aware of your efforts than anyone else—are *least* likely to give yourself the good feedback you deserve.

Now that you're aware of the importance of appropriate, adaptive monologues, what can you do to improve yours? A three-step strategy, if practiced diligently, may be very helpful in cleaning up some of your negative self-statements.

The first step is to detect the occurrence of both inappropriate and appropriate thoughts. This may not be quite as simple as it sounds. If you're like many people, you may go through an entire day without monitoring what you say to yourself. This doesn't mean that your thoughts are unconscious—only that you seldom make an effort to listen in on them. Getting in the habit of tuning in to your thoughts is the first step in modifying them. One technique for developing this skill is to perform a mental inventory whenever you feel tempted, discouraged, or depressed. Go over what you've been thinking for the last few minutes. Have you been making excuses, labeling yourself a martyr, or criticizing yourself?

Once you have detected the cognitive culprit, evaluate its reasonableness. Are you catastrophizing? Are you turning a behavioral deficiency into a personal inadequacy? What would you say to someone else in this situation?

When you have pinpointed the problematical self-statements and evaluated their reasonableness (for example, "I'm depressed because I only lost half a pound last week—that's silly, it took several years to put these pounds on. Besides I need to be thinking *behavior*, not pounds."), then say something encouraging to yourself. "I'm making progress, slowly but surely—a couple of months from now I'll laugh at how I almost sabotaged my own success."

Detect; evaluate; encourage. This three-step sequence, with practice, may prove to be a valuable aid in modifying your problematical monologues. The following table shows some categories of problem thoughts which often occur during attempts to change eating habits. Adaptive monologues which should be developed regarding each of the problem categories are also listed. Do any of these sound familiar to you? You probably can also come up with some of your own. There are, of course, many other categories and possible solutions. Your mental inventory will reveal patterns of self-talk that are unique to you. Whatever the specific content of your private monologues, it can be modified. Remember: detect, evaluate, encourage.

You may recall that our discussion of your cognitive ecology began by pointing out three ideas: you, as a human being, think a lot; your thoughts influence your behavior and your feelings; and you can learn to control what you think about. You have learned that two categories of thoughts that often require remediation are your personal goals and your private monologues. Guidelines for setting more reasonable goals have been suggested; strategies for improving your private monologues have been presented.

Your cognitive "digestive" system may well feel a bit overloaded; you should expect this temporarily—and talk to yourself ap-

TABLE 3

Problem Category	Negative Monologues	Appropriate Monologues
Pounds lost	"I'm not losing fast enough." "I've starved myself and haven't lost a thing." "I've been more consistent than Mary and she is losing faster than I am—it's not fair."	"Pounds don't count; if I continue my eating habits, the pounds will be lost." "Have patience—those pounds took a long time to get there. As long as they stay off permanently, I'll settle for any progress." "It takes a while to break down fat and absorb the extra water produced. I'm not going to worry about it."
Capabilities	"I just don't have the will power." "I'm just naturally fat." "Why should this work— nothing else has." "I'll probably just regain it." "What the heck—I'd rather be fat than miserable; besides I'm not *that* heavy."	"There's no such thing as 'will power'—just poor planning. If I make a few improvements here and there and take things one day at a time, I can be very successful." "It's going to be nice to be permanently rid of all this extra baggage—I'm starting to feel better already."
Excuses	"If it weren't for my job and the kids, I could lose weight." "It's just impossible to eat right with a schedule like mine."	"My schedule isn't any worse than anyone else's. What I need to do is be a bit more creative in how to improve my eating." "Eating doesn't satisfy psy-

propriately. Cleaning up your cognitive ecology will demand time and energy; it requires careful planning and persistent effort over a period of months. The most adaptive thing you can say to yourself about it is—it's worth it! The dividends in terms of changed behavior, positive feelings, and long-term motivation are virtually immeasurable. Whatever the specific behavior you are attempting to change, your thoughts, specifically your goals and self-statements, will play a major role in your success or failure. Good cognitive ecology is an *essential* in personal science.

Problem Category	Negative Monologues	Appropriate Monologues
	"I'm just so nervous all the time—I have to eat to satisfy my psychological needs." "Maybe next time . . . ."	chological problems—it creates them." "Job, kids, or whatever, I'm the one in control."
Goals	"Well, there goes my diet. That coffee cake probably cost me two pounds, and after I promised myself— no more sweets." "I always blow it on the weekends." Fine—I start the day off with a doughnut. I may as well enjoy myself today."	"What is this—the Olympics? I don't need perfect habits, just improved ones." "Why should one sweet or an extra portion blow it for me? I'll cut back elsewhere." "Those high standards are unrealistic." "Fantastic—I had a small piece of cake and it didn't blow the day."
Food thoughts	"I can't stop thinking about sweets." "I had images of cakes and pies all afternoon—it must mean that I need sugar." "When we order food at a restaurant, I continue thinking about what I have ordered until it arrives."	"Whenever I find myself thinking about food, I quickly change the topic to some other pleasant experience." "If I see a magazine ad or commercial for food and I start thinking about it, I distract my attention by doing something else (phoning a friend, getting the mail, etc.)."

ILLUSTRATION

Miss Jones was a 25-year-old elementary school teacher who had picked up three or four pounds a year since her college days. A survey of her eating habits suggested that her sweet tooth was getting her into trouble. Her second graders frequently included her in their snack-time treats. She also noticed that afternoon pick-me-ups were usually cookies or chips. Late evening snacking also emphasized sweets.

Having unsuccessfully tried cutting back several times in the past, Miss Jones decided to make an all-out effort to shape up her eating habits by eliminating sweets from her diet. She cleared out her cookie jar at home and announced to her friends that she was going on a diet. Feeling quite virtuous, she started off her week with high hopes. During the first three days of her diet, she was perfect; not a single violation marred her record. However, she noted that instead of seeming *less* important, sweets seemed to be becoming *more* important. She caught herself staring enviously at some of her skinny students as they munched candy bars and cookies. She began to feel like a martyr, resentful and angry at the unfairness of it all. Furthermore, after four days of depriving herself, she hadn't lost an ounce!

Then came Friday—and her favorite student's birthday. Miss Jones had been invited to his birthday party. David's mother had assured her that the invitation was a real compliment; David had disliked each of his teachers in the past. Not only was he doing better school work this year; he wanted her to attend his party. Her typical enthusiasm for such an occasion was spoiled all day by anticipating the cake, ice cream, and other treats she knew she would encounter. She found herself actually dreading the party, and resentful of the invitation. She stubbornly refused her piece of cake, determined to stick it out—and drove home hungry, frustrated, and miserable. She had survived it—and for what? It had spoiled her week, her day, and the party. How many more days would this have to go on before she lost enough weight?

A few minutes later Miss Jones was in the bakery section of the supermarket, stocking up on sweets for the weekend. After an initial surge of relief at satisfying her craving for sweets, she spent a miserable weekend criticizing herself and feeling depressed and hopeless about her fat future.

That sequence may sound very familiar. Now, let's turn Miss Jones into a personal scientist and see what she would do at this point.

Stage 1: Specify area. After learning about the significant impact of one's private environment upon behavior and feelings, Miss Jones decided to minitor her food-related thoughts to see if they were maladaptive and self-defeating.

Stage 2: Collect data. On a small card she recorded all of her food-related thoughts and the time of day they occurred. Her data for the third day are shown below.

TABLE 4

Time	Thoughts
7:30	"I'd really like a doughnut but I'm not going to blow my day."
8:15	"It's not fair; I'm really trying and I haven't lost anything."
9:10	"Wish I had a doughnut or something; I'm hungry."
10:00	"It's not fair; it's snack time and all I get is water."
11:30	"Nothing tastes as good when I know there's no dessert."
12:10	"Look at them; they stuff themselves with sweets and stay skinny."
1:15	"Maybe I could have just a couple of cookies after school. I've earned them."
2:30	"Look at them—running off to their afternoon snacks. It's not fair."
3:15	"I don't care if I'm fat; I'll never lose anyway. It's not worth it."
4:30	"I might as well eat and enjoy it. I'll never be thin, no matter what I do."
5:45	"You pig. Now you feel stuffed and you've ruined your day."
7:30	"What a failure I am. I don't deserve to be thin."
9:00	"I'll never learn, will I? It's no use."
10:30	"I feel hopeless. I've tried everything and I always blow it."

Notice that Miss Jones monitored only her food-related thoughts and the time they occurred. It might have been helpful to record what happened right before each food thought. This might have revealed some cues for her thoughts, thus warning her about especially difficult occasions or times of day.

Stage 3: Identify patterns. Despite the difficulty of recording thoughts and the possible incompleteness of her record keeping, some problematical patterns were very obvious. Miss Jones noted that nearly 100 percent of her food thoughts were inappropriate and self-defeating. They seemed to fall into several categories: pounds lost, traits, excuses, and dire predictions—predictions about her fat future. A second pattern that was readily apparent was that many of these thoughts seemed to be a reaction to a goal that was too perfectionistic— complete abstinence from sweets.

Stage 4: Examine options. Miss Jones specified the following options as possible solutions:

   a.   try to distract from food thoughts;
   b.   modify the goal of eliminating sweets;
   c.   change her maladaptive thoughts.

Stage 5: Narrow and experiment. Distraction from food thoughts seemed to be a feasible partial solution; she could quite easily call a friend or go for a walk to avoid eating. However, the frequency of maladaptive thoughts suggested that it would not be sufficient, especially in the presence of sweets. Miss Jones decided to try the other two solutions: to modify her goal, and to change her maladaptive thoughts by the three-step strategy: detection, evaluation, and replacement. Her first step was to modify her goal of *no* sweets to a goal of one per day for one week. Each day that she achieved that goal, she praised herself specifically for setting and achieving a reasonable goal. Her second step was to cue herself to tune in to her inappropriate thoughts. She placed a small piece of adhesive tape on the face of her watch and on clocks at home. Each time she checked the time, she also checked her thoughts. She did a quick inventory of her thoughts for the preceding few minutes. Each time she pinpointed a problematical self-statement or food thought, she evaluated it and replaced it with a more appropriate, encouraging one. She made a special effort to stop long enough after finishing the sequence to praise herself for completing it.

Stage 6: Compare data. Miss Jones found that more reasonable goal setting and the detection-evaluation-replacement sequence had a significant impact on her thoughts. Her data showed an impressive decrease in negative self-statements and inappropriate thoughts (pounds, etc.) and a dramatic increase in positive self-statements and appropriate thoughts. She noted also an uneven improvement in her feelings; on some days she seemed to feel better about herself and more optimistic about her future eating habits.

Stage 7: Extend, revise, or replace. Miss Jones felt very satisfied with the results of her solutions. She decided to continue them, but with two modifications. She had noticed that often she would detect a maladaptive thought and then criticize herself for thinking it, rather than replacing it with something more encouraging. Consequently, she revised her strategy so that when she detected a problematical thought, she would write down on a card an appropriate one to replace it. Actually writing down appropriate thoughts would force her to think straight.

Her second revision involved changing her cue. The pieces of tape on her watch and clock were becoming so familiar she hardly noticed them; as a result, their helpfulness as cues was diminishing. She decided to increase the efficiency of her cueing system by replacing the pieces of tape with trading stamps and to extend it by placing stamps on all the mirrors in the house, as well as on the bathroom scale.

Remembering that learning to think more adaptively takes time, and that corresponding change in feelings may be uneven or delayed, Miss Jones decided to continue her program for a minimum of another three weeks.

ASSIGNMENT 1

Since you have not yet learned about some of the specific behaviors involved in changing eating habits, you will not be asked to work on goal setting in this assignment. Later chapters will provide ample opportunities for you to apply your knowledge from this chapter to setting reasonable, flexible goals.

Right now you are expected to focus on learning to tune in to your food-related thoughts. For at least one week (and you are strongly encouraged to continue it through the next couple of assignments, or longer), you are to imitate Miss Jones. You will need trading stamps and small cards. Place the stamps, as she did, on your watch, clocks, mirrors, and your scale. Also place one in a prominent place in your purse or wallet, and carry a couple of cards with you at all times.

Each time you see a stamp, stop and review your thoughts for the preceding few minutes. Can you find any appropriate ones? If so, stop and praise yourself for constructive thinking. What about maladaptive ones? Have you been thinking about (or imaging) tempting foods? Have you thought about pounds or traits or made excuses to yourself? Have you been self-critical?

Concentrate on evaluating each of these thoughts in terms of what you've learned in this chapter. Try to be specific in your evaluation. *What* is unreasonable about that thought?

Now, write down an encouraging replacement for it on one of your cards—and think about it for a few moments. Now, praise yourself for completing the sequence.

Remember to change your cue if it becomes so familiar you start to ignore it. Also remember that it takes practice to become efficient at listening in on your own thoughts. If you detect few food thoughts the first few days, it probably reflects the newness of your efforts rather than a low frequency of food thoughts.

Your cognitive ecology will have an impact on the effort you expend and the success you achieve in later assignments. To increase your positive returns and to maintain your motivation, it should be considered an ongoing assignment.

7
Engineering
a Slim Environment

You have now learned the personal science sequence—the steps in successful self-control. You have learned about one of the elements that is crucial to the successful application of this sequence, whatever the nature of the particular patterns you wish to change. Good cognitive ecology is important, regardless of the type of pattern you are trying to improve. It is just as essential to changing work habits or study habits—or any others—as it is to modifying eating patterns. Now you are ready to focus on a second element that is essential in weight control. You are ready to learn about another factor that is critically important in self-control—regardless of the topic. This second factor is environmental engineering.

SUCCESSFUL SELF-CONTROL
INVOLVES EFFECTIVE
ENVIRONMENTAL ENGINEERING

Successful weight controllers live in "slender" environments; they are experts in environmental design. The importance of this element, like that of cognitive ecology, cannot be overemphasized. If you want to become more skilled in self-control, you must become more proficient in environmental planning. If you want to become a successful weight watcher, you must become an efficient environmental designer.

Now just what are we talking about here? Engineers are familiar enough figures in our modern world. They are our professional planners. Their efforts improve our environment in countless ways. Most of us can think of hundreds of ways in which they make our world a safer and more pleasant place to live. Environmental engineering to most of us means planning cities and building bridges. This term may sound quite unfamiliar, or even strange, however, when applied to the area of weight control. Environmental engineering or designing is a task for an engineer, or a scientist, isn't it? Yes, it is. And that's just the point. You are becoming a scientist—a personal scientist. To do so, you must become an engineer.

If environmental planning or engineering is such an important element in self-control, why does it sound so strange to most weight watchers? One answer is that it runs directly contrary to the old notion of "will power." The will power concept nourishes a culturally prevalent myth of autonomy: namely, that people are completely independent agents, little influenced by their surroundings. People in our culture are taught that habit change is simply a matter of "making up your mind." Many of us are victims of the false notion that behavior is influenced only by inborn forces beyond our control. And "will power" is usually at the top of that list. Thoughts and goals *are* important factors in self-control, as we have seen, but they are not the only factors.

Your actions *are* influenced by your environment—every day of your life. Further, they are influenced by several environments, not just one. The power of environmental influence becomes more obvious when you realize that you are the recipient of at least three sources of input from your surroundings: cognitive, physical, and social. Each has an important impact on your behavior. First, your own *cognitions* may exert a considerable influence on the way you feel and the way you act. Your own thoughts, monologues, goals, and standards constitute your private environment. This is, in one sense, your most personal environment; you are the only person who has access to its contents.

Second, your behavior is influenced by your *physical* environment. Sensitivity to your physical surroundings is literally essential to your survival. You are constantly perceiving and interpreting information that tells you how to behave in a given situation. That stoplight on the corner is a familiar example of a physical cue that influences your behavior. It is one example among hundreds which you encounter and respond to every day.

Third, your actions are significantly influenced by your *social* environment—the actions of other people toward you. You constantly receive questions, instructions, requests, advice, praise, criticism (the list goes on and on) which affect your behavior in a variety of ways. A high percentage of your daily behavior occurs in direct response to someone else's behavior, or in anticipation of someone else's feedback.

The point is: *you do not live in a vacuum.* A truly vast experimental literature documents the continuous and important impact of environmental influence on your behavior, an influence that cannot be overlooked in the development of self-control skills. In fact, understanding the relationship between behavior and environment may be considered the ABCs of self-control. A helpful way to consider this interaction is to think of a *behavior* as being sandwiched between two events: an *antecedent* and a *consequence.* Your behavior is *preceded* by some event (an antecedent event, or cue), and *followed* by some event (a consequence); each of these events may significantly affect the behavior that occurs between them. Your eating behavior is no exception to this pattern. Try to think of some of the antecedent events that serve as cues for your eating. Remember, these may come from any of your environments. Consider your physical environment, for example. Many physical objects or situations may serve as powerful eating cues. It has been demonstrated tht the physical presence of food is one of the strongest such cues. How many times have you said, between mouthfuls, "I don't even want this"? Yet you eat it—simply because it's there. Another powerful physical cue is so familiar you may be unaware of its influence—the clock! Many individuals eat because they think it's *time* to eat. They let the clock, rather than appetite, dictate their eating behavior. They eat because food is there or because it's mealtime, rather than because they are hungry. They eat in response to their external, rather than internal, physical environment.

What about your cognitive environment: What thoughts lead you to the kitchen? Many times, simply thinking of food is enough to get you there. Self-defeating goals and monologues, as we've seen, may actually encourage you to eat. Finally, consider your social environment. How often do you eat in response to cues from those around you? How many times do you eat because someone else is eating? How often do you go to lunch because everyone else is going? How many times do your family or friends *offer* you food, or encourage you to eat? ("Oh, go ahead; one piece of pie won't hurt you.")

You are bombarded with food cues from each of your environments, probably much more frequently than you realize. You may have *learned* to eat in response to a variety of events, rather than to physiological hunger.

This is only half the story. Environmental *consequences* also influence eating. And, again, these may be physical, cognitive, or social. One of the strongest consequences of eating is physical; food tastes good. When you eat, you *immediately* experience positive results. You receive an immediate reward. The positive consequences of weight control are long-term, not immediate. These long-term consequences may sometimes be outweighed by the immediate and pleasant consequences of food consumption, which are a frequent factor in overeating. Ironically, however, *over*eating is frequently followed by self-punishing statements, which may actually encourage you to eat again. ("Oh, what's the use. I'll never make it.") Your social environment is also a very important source of feedback. Inappropriate reassurances ("It's all right; you just can't help it.") *or* severe criticism ("Well, you pigged out again.") may increase overeating. Social feedback, often given with the best of intentions, often plays an important role in maintaining maladaptive eating patterns.

The ABCs of self-control suggest that behavior is not autonomous; it is influenced daily by an enormous variety of cues and consequences. Now, does this mean you are a victim of environmental circumstances, controlled by external influences? The answer to that question is an emphatic *no*. *You* influence your environments, just as they influence you. The relationship between your environments and your behavior is a reciprocal one; it is a two-way street. Self-control is an active process; you are an active agent in creating and designing your environments—whether you are aware of it or not. *You* can influence your environment to work for or against you; you can create a slim environment as well as a fat one. You can become an effective environmental engineer.

The basic skill in environmental engineering is changing the cues and consequences that encourage faulty eating habits to those that encourage good eating habits. You can program your eating environments in two helpful ways: by *increasing* cues and consequences that facilitate appropriate patterns and by *decreasing* those that encourage inappropriate patterns. What people or places, thoughts or things encourage you to eat inappropriately? What could you do to get those influences to work for, not against, you?

In the last chapter you learned some ways to improve your cognitive ecology by setting reasonable goals and cleaning up your self-statements. Remember your private world is your most personal *and* your most permanent one. Your physical surroundings may change; friends come and go over the years. But your cognitive environment will be with you for the rest of your life. As you have already learned, it can be your worst enemy or your most staunch and stable ally.

In the remainder of this book you will be learning how to change your physical environment to help you eat *and* exercise wisely. Let's focus now on your social environment and see how you can redesign it for a slimmer, healthier you.

GUIDELINES FOR BECOMING A SOCIAL ENGINEER

First, what is your social environment? How does it affect you? How important is it in your weight control endeavors? Your social environment consists, very simply, of your interactions with people around you. The prominent figures in your social surroundings are your family and close friends; however, your coworkers, neighbors, and even casual acquaintances may also play a significant role. These familiar individuals are important to you in more ways than one. Many of them are people you love and value; you are probably well aware of their importance in this regard. They are important to you in another way which may be masked by daily familiarity: their behavior exerts a powerful influence on your own.

First, as we have seen, they may cue you, directly or indirectly, to behave in certain ways. Often the cue is direct. You are probably a frequent recipient of requests and advice. How often do you hear: "Would you mind doing this for me?" or "This is what I think you should do." Possibly too often! People, especially family members, are notorious for making demands and giving advice, wanted or not. The cue may also be indirect; merely observing someone else doing something may lead to your performing the same activity. Human beings are great imitators; that is a scientific statement as well as an age-old observation!

Second, your social life is a source of feedback. Other people not only cue you to act in certain ways; they present consequences when you do! Feedback from others can exert a powerful influence on your behavior; your weight control efforts are no exception. Let's consider your probable response to different types of social consequences. Assume you are working hard at improving your eating habits. Now, imagine your reactions to three types of feedback. Suppose you receive *no* feedback. No one shows an interest in your efforts or your results. Would you continue them? For how long? Now, visualize comments from your loved ones such as: "You look great"; "You're really trying hard"; "I'm so proud of you." How does positive feedback, or praise, from others affect your efforts? Finally, think about hearing statements such as "Why don't you give up? You never stick to anything, anyway!" How do you react to criticism for your efforts?

Several factors affect your responses to feedback from others; you don't always respond in the same way. The importance of the person giving the feedback may make a difference; for example, a spouse's feedback may have more impact than a neighbor's. Many other factors are also important. For example, you may ignore criticism from others when you think it is undeserved. In this case, your own self-evaluation should be most important. Generally speaking, however, you are most likely to maintain your weight control efforts in a supportive social environment; you are less likely to continue them in neutral or critical social surroundings. In fact, some recent evidence suggests that social support may be one of the most essential factors in successful weight control. Food, in our culture, is very much a social commodity. Much of your interaction with your family involves food. A high percentage of your family's time together may be spent at the kitchen table, or snacking in front of the T.V. Mealtime is the only "together" time for many families. Much of your contact with your broader social group also emphasizes food. Entertainment often focuses upon food. Dinner parties, brunches, luncheons, desserts, cookouts, picnics, coffees— these are but a few examples. Very rarely does entertainment or recreation *exclude* food.

Your social environment does influence your eating habits; it provides specific cues and consequences in addition to a general cultural focus upon food. So far, however, we have only looked at half the picture. You, also, are a social agent. You, also, provide cues and consequences which influence the behavior of others. You can use your own social influence to elicit *helpful* cues and consequences which will facilitate your weight control endeavor. You can establish a supportive social environment which works *for* you, not against you. You can become a successful social engineer.

How can you get the social support you need? Let's start with family and friends.

Family and Friends' Support

Friends and family members hold a prime position of social influence, for at least two reasons. First, they're often (though not always) the individuals with whom you spend a great deal of your time. Second, as loved ones, they are usually the individuals you most want to please. If you are the family cook, you influence very directly what your family members eat. More subtly, they also influence *what* you eat—and *how much* and *how often*. What, when, how much, and how frequently do *your* family members eat? The answers to these questions often are a good index of your own eating patterns.

What is your eating atmosphere at home? Some weight watchers are fortunate enough to live with individuals who are good social supporters; others may live with individuals who have good eating habits of their own. Some weight watchers are extremely fortunate; their family members do both. They encourage weight control by modeling good habits *and* by giving extensive and appropriate social support. Maybe you live with such saints. If you do, you are lucky—and unusual. Most overweight individuals do not live in this kind of environment. If excessive weight has been a long-term worry, if you have tried and tried again, it is very likely that some of the following social patterns apply to your home and/or your friends:

Pattern 1. Loved ones often tease about weight problems and criticize you for overeating. Attemps at improvement are often the brunt of jokes and severe pessimism. How often do you hear statements like: "Well, here she goes again"; or "I've heard this before; what diet is it *this* time?" Discouraging, aren't they?

Pattern 2. Friends and family openly discourage and sabotage your efforts by offering high calorie treats. Reasons for this type of nonsupport may range from financial to psychological. Occasionally the culprit may himself (or herself) be overweight and feel pressured to reduce if his spouse is successful.

Pattern 3. Family or friends simply ignore your efforts. They seem oblivious to your conscientious attempts and are pessimistic about your success.

Pattern 4. Loved ones verbally encourage your weight control efforts but frequently impede success by requesting high calorie snacks, offering you food, or using food (for example, candy or pastry) as a token of affection. It is not uncommon for individuals in this pattern to praise initial weight losses but then ignore successful maintenance.

Do any of these patterns strike home? If any of them are prevalent, you should take specific steps to redesign your social environment.

1. *Request family's and friends' active involvement in your weight control efforts.* Your first engineering task is to ask your loved ones' assistance specifically and sincerely. Incidentally, that includes the kids. Carefully explain the personal science sequence as an effective way to self-control. Remember that their initial response may be in terms of "another diet"; it is crucially important that they understand the differences between your past attempts at dieting and the personal science approach. Be sure to explain the emphasis on patterns versus pounds. Also explain that this approach emphasizes gradual changes and does not encourage the elimination of entire categories of food. This will encourage reasonable standards on their part and should avoid a critical reaction when they see you enjoying occasional sweets. Describe to them the important influence they exert on your eating and exercise patterns; let them know you need and will actively appreciate their support. Request, don't demand. Ideally, one or more of your family members, or even close friends, will agree to read along with you. That would guarantee a clearer understanding of your attempts and the principles underlying them. If that is not a feasible alternative, be as thorough and sincere as possible in explaining both the self-control approach and your need for their assistance. Try to anticipate their questions and be prepared to answer them.

Let's deal with some problems you may encounter in asking for assistance from others. Some people find it difficult to seek support from others—even their families or close friends. These are usually the same individuals who perceive, or want to perceive, themselves as completely independent, autonomous human beings. They want to do it on their own; they consider it a sign of weakness or dependence to ask for support. If this description fits you, remember that you are not asking your loved ones to to *start* influencing you. They already influence you—one way or another. You are taking the initiative by asking them to influence you in particular ways, to utilize their influence to help rather than hinder your efforts. It may be helpful for a moment to swap roles with your spouse, friend, son, or daughter. If he (or she) were the weight controller, and you were the family member or friend, would you want to help? Would you want to know specifically just *how* to help? Lack of social support often stems from lack of information or understanding, rather than from lack of concern.

2. Rearrange family's and friends' reactions to your eating habits and weight control attempts. Begin by requesting that they not tease or criticize you about weight loss or overeating. Your efforts to improve should not be the brunt of jokes, even when they are meant affectionately. Neither should your attempts be the target of criticism. Sarcasm and critical remarks are the last thing you need. It should not be your loved ones' job to police you. Instead, ask them to praise you for progress. Their motto should be: if you can't say something good, then don't say anything at all. Emphasize that their praise is very important to you; assure them that it will greatly facilitate your progress. You don't have to lose weight for them to express praise. Tell them to set their standards modestly and to provide you with frequent reminders that they appreciate your efforts. Ask that they remember you are aiming for improvement, not perfection, and that you are working on patterns, not pounds. Don't encourage questions about what you weigh, but rather what you have done. Be prepared: it may take some time for them to get into the habit of recognizing and applauding your appropriate eating patterns. This is because some appropriate behaviors involve *not* performing an undesirable act (preferably by replacing it with a more appropriate one) and may be harder to detect. Tell them specifically what behaviors you are trying to increase; tell them which less desirable behaviors you are trying to replace. Again, their feedback should accentuate the positive and they should not be critical or make you feel guilty when you slip. You can be instrumental in hastening your family's development of appropriate reactions by giving them gentle feedback, discussing your progress, and providing them with generous appreciation for their supportive efforts.

3. *Request the cooperation of family and friends in reducing your exposure to food.* At this point you should understand why you want to make foods less available or conspicuous. You want to change the focus on food in your environment in as many ways as possible. The following is one of the most important and successful ways of changing eating habits: *request that your spouse, children, and friends not offer you food* (either during or between meals). Many people are amazed at the quantity of food they consume simply because a loved one has offered it. Unfortunately, offering one's spouse the last biscuit at a meal or sharing a midnight snack is sometimes mistakenly perceived as a sign of affection. This pattern is a very dangerous one. If your spouse (or other family member) is overweight and would like to reduce, make the pact a mutual one.

The significance of this one very simple but powerful strategy should not be underestimated. You may be surprised at the frequency with which you catch yourself being offered food. An auxiliary to this suggestion deals with keeping food around the house. Ideally, your family will cooperate in not buying high calorie presents or bringing home sweets. However, if they insist on having snacks in the house, request that they be stored inconspicuously, and that family members serve themselves (without offering you any, of course). Ask also that they choose snacks that *you* dislike.

Also request their cooperation in the foods they will accept at meals. If your family is accustomed to eating a variety of foods, this may be easy to accomplish. If they are strictly the meat and potatoes type, if your family's daily menus strongly emphasize carbohydrates and fats, you may have to be a more careful engineer. Give ample assurance that you're *not* requesting drastic changes such as giving up desserts entirely. Assure them that you're asking for a gradual shift in emphasis to lower calorie, and probably more nutritious, foods.

Finally, ask their help in reducing the general focus on food in your lives—for example, its importance in your conversations or entertainment. Discussions of food should be decreased; they frequently lead to snacking. Similarly, de-emphasize the role of eating in celebrations and evenings out. A movie or a play can be used as a nonfattening way of celebrating a birthday, anniversary, etc. Friends or relatives can be entertained in your home without being deluged by chips, dips, and desserts. Recipes for *good* lower calorie treats are available (for example, carob cake, sugarless plum cake). Raw vegetables can be substituted for chips and crackers. Notice, we are saying "reduce, decrease, de-emphasize"—not eliminate! We are *not* suggesting radical changes in your family's eating lifestyle. Be sure that this important point is very clear to them.

4. *Request interest and cooperation in the development of a more active lifestyle.* In a later chapter you will learn more about the value of a more active life. Exercise plays a crucially important role in weight control and good health. Your establishment and maintenance of an active daily routine will be enhanced if your family will participate. If that option is not available, ask them at least to express an interest in your attempts to become more active.

5. *Remember your role as a social influencer.* The importance of this final guideline cannot be overemphasized. In all of the above suggestions you are requesting the assistance and cooperation of family and friends. Whether you receive it is very largely determined by *you*. *You* are the person in the key position; you are the person who knows what you need from your loved ones. You should now know how to increase the likelihood that you'll receive it. You are asking for their support because you realize that it can have a major and helpful effect on your behavior—specifically, your eating behavior. *Your most important task as a social engineer may well be your support of their support!* Remember, their behavior is as dependent on *your* cues and consequences as yours is on theirs. Reward them generously for *any* attempt to cooperate or to encourage you. Thank them sincerely for their praise; let them know that you notice and appreciate it.

After your initial explanation of the self-control approach and your general request for assistance, keep family and friends specifically informed of what you are working on each week. Tell them explicitly what you need praise *for*. And, by all means, inform them of you progress. Let them share in your successes; let them know those successes are partly the result of *their* efforts. Finally, beware of a frequent tendency to discredit your loved ones' praise. Some individuals ask for their family's support; then, when they receive it, they put it down or argue that it is not deserved (because it was requested, because their loved ones didn't see them snacking earlier, etc.). If your family and friends value you and your efforts, their feedback is not artificial or insincere, regardless of whether it was requested. It takes time for families to change their interaction patterns; there is nothing illegal about priming the pump to facilitate those changes.

Now, let's do some troubleshooting. Good engineers try to anticipate and head off problems before they begin. Let's consider some problems which you might encounter.

What do you do if they do not approve of your weight reduction efforts? The first question to ask yourself is: do they have some justification? *Are* you really overweight? Is your goal a healthy weight for you, or emaciation? Is your weight problem really a flab problem? Would some firming up take care of it? If you are the *only* person you know who thinks you need to lose weight, you may be better off to lower your standards than your weight.

If there is little question of your need to reduce, examine possible reasons for their disapproval. Are *they* overweight? Do they feel pressured by your efforts? If this is the case, it is imperative that you be extremely sensitive to their feelings and perceptions. Even indirect cues from you that they should be also reducing will almost certainly sabotage your efforts to obtain their support. In this particular situation, tact and praise are most effective; pressure and criticism are least effective.

Another possible reason for their disapproval may be their memories of your past attempts to lose weight. If they have suffered through a series of your fad diets—and suffered from your fatigue and crabbiness in the process—they may be very leery of your current attempt. If this is the problem, and if you can convince them that this approach is different, you should be able to win their support.

What do you do if your loved ones approve of your weight control project but will not actively cooperate? First, ask yourself if you are expecting too much too soon. Patterns change slowly, with persistent effort. Just as you are asking them to support gradual changes in your patterns, you should support gradual changes in *their* behaviors. Are *you* tuned in to their efforts, or are you overlooking some small steps they are taking in the right direction? Check your standards before proceeding.

If you are very confident of their lack of support, sit down and consider your loved ones as individuals. What approach could you take that might work with them, considering *their* personal needs? Try to analyze what factors are prohibiting their support. Do they have enough information about the personal science sequence, about your specific goals and needs? Have you clearly communicated your needs to them in a positive, loving way? Are they taking you seriously? Are they pessimistic about your success? Is it a lack of concern, or lack of awareness, on their part that is prohibiting their support?

Spend some time considering your family and friends as unique individuals. Try to step into their shoes and to figure out how they view your efforts. *Then* choose an option.

Now, what if you have tried everything you can think of to win their support—to no avail? Some families, for a variety of reasons, do refuse to support weight watchers' efforts and seem immune to change. If this is the case, success may be more difficult to achieve, but it is not impossible by any means. If family support is not forthcoming, you still have other forms of support; you can concentrate on improving your other environments (physical and cognitive) and on increasing social support from outside your family. Each of these environments is extremely important in your success. It is fortunate, however, that there are several. One advantage of a wide base of support is that when one aspect fails you can rely more heavily on others.

Group Support

A support source that you may want to consider is that of a formal group—a group formed explicitly for the purpose of facilitating weight control attempts. Such a group can be a valuable replacement for or addition to your family support base. A small group of friends or acquaintances who share your interest in becoming a better problem solver can be a valuable source of assistance and feedback. The sharing of ideas and the encouragement provided by such a group may be especially helpful if other aspects of your social environment are weak.

Consider this possibility with one recommendation clearly in mind: a good group is helpful but not essential; a bad group is catastrophic. *No* group is better than a bad group. Your individual development as a problem solver may actually be harmed by group gimmicks or social sympathy. If you can form a group of interested, concerned people—interested in realistic and reasonable ways to change eating patterns, and concerned about each other's progress as well as their own—then go ahead. We urge that you pursue this alternative *only* under these conditions.

One other word of caution. It is very easy to let group support become your sole, or even primary, support. It should be neither of these—unless you plan to continue it for the rest of your life. Remember, you are trying to establish patterns you can live with forever. A group may be very helpful initially, but it is a temporary measure. Becoming overly dependent on it will deter, not facilitate, your development as an independent self-controller. We strongly urge you to keep these considerations in mind.

Now let's look at some guidelines for establishing effective groups.

1. *Planning: Keep your eye on the brass ring.* Plan your group with your purpose clearly in mind. Each member should be clearly committed to the self-control, personal science approach. Your purpose should be very explicitly and mutually defined as providing support in the development of the skills this approach suggests.

2. *Admissions: Eliminate the dead weight.* The composition of the group should conform to your purpose. This is not a bridge club, so be rigid about your admission policy. First, group members should be friends with whom you can be honest, friends who feel mutually comfortable to discuss problems openly, without embarrassment. Second, group members should be motivated; if you have to talk them into it, don't! Each member must be individually and personally motivated so that he or she can be a giving as well as taking participant in the group. Each person must be so motivated that he or she plans to pursue this approach—group or no group! Third, group members should be friends, not rivals. Petty jealousies, secret satisfaction at others' failures, subtle put-downs—these are disastrous to both group and individual success. Participants should be genuinely concerned individuals who can give honest but genuinely *supportive* feedback. Finally, avoid deadweight members—hangers-on. Very frequently, people express an interest in the group's purpose, when in reality they have purposes of their own. They may be bored or lonely, looking for companionship rather than progress. The old saying, "misery loves company," is *not* appropriate for a problem solving group. Success and support, *not* sympathy, should be each person's goal. It is sometimes difficult to say no to a friend who falls into this category. Be tactful, but be firm. It is a disservice to you, to the group, *and* to the person involved, to allow him in the group. Our experience strongly suggests that it is not only more effective, but kinder in the long run, to exclude this type of individual from the group. It is better to meet this person's need for friendship by some other means.

3. *Mutual Support: Praise appropriately.* Group interaction should emphasize honesty, perseverance and support. There is a difference between flattery and deserved praise. Positive feedback should be given for progress and effort—not for excuses. Don't encourage patterns of buck passing and idle resolutions. On the other hand, members should not be perfectionistic in their praise giving; small steps should be warmly supported. Effort, not success, is the watchword. There is a real difference, however, between praising effort and excuses. It is easy for a person's effort to deteriorate into meaningless confessions and lame excuses, especially when these are met by condolences from the rest of the group. It is easy to fall into a pattern of calling other members to gossip and giggle about failures. Sympathy may feel good—but it isn't helpful. If someone in the group is not doing well, he needs problem-solving assistance, not excuses. The truly helpful group member is sensitive to and supportive of others' efforts, but kindly intolerant of excuses and sympathy seeking.

Group members may be valuable assistants in goal setting and problem solving as well as sources of support. A good example is their potential role in the establishment and supervision of *behavioral contracts*. As a personal scientist you will be setting many goals for behavior change; a behavioral contract is a means of specifying and formalizing your goals. In drawing up such a contract you are basically committing yourself to something in writing. A contract consists of two parts. First, it specifies what you will do by *when*. The desired behavior should be spelled out in detail (for example, "I will buy *only* 2 percent milk and low calorie soda during the next seven days"). Second, your contract should specify a reward you will earn by performing the stated behavior (for example, "I will buy myself a pair of earrings on April 12 if I have achieved my goal").

BEHAVIORAL CONTRACT

Name _____   Date _____

Agreement: During the next _____ days, if I successfully (specify desired behavior)

_____

then I will reward myself with (specify reward) _____

_____

I will be consistent in rewarding myself if I perform the above specified behaviors and I will not reward myself if I don't perform them. If earned, my self-reward will be received before (date) _____

                                          Signature _____
Witness _____

Witness: Please contact the above person on or before the self-reward date to determine
whether (a) the desired behavior was successfully performed, and (b) the self-
reward was appropriately administered. Your encouragement of consistency
and persistence will be appreciated.

FIGURE 2

Such a behavioral or self-reward contract has several advantages. It states precisely what you will do and what you will receive, and it does so in a formal and public way. Both of these increase your probability of success. We suggest that you ask a group member to review your contract and to witness it. This will provide an opportunity for feedback on the reasonableness of your goal and reward; it will also enhance the likelihood that you will follow through.

The contract conditions should be realistic and fair. Generally, the chosen goal should be attainable about 80 percent of the time, so that the emphasis is positive—you are usually successful in earning your self-reward. The agreement conditions can be *gradually* made more difficult. Earned self-rewards should be presented immediately after (never before) the attainment of the desired performance. Frequent small rewards are preferable to large delayed ones. A self-reward period should not extend beyond one to two weeks.

Finally, a successful self-reward system must satisfy several conditions. First of all, it must involve a consistent "if-then" system. For example, "If I limit my eating to mealtimes for the next week, I will buy myself a record album." This means that if you are successful, you must comply with the agreement and immediately buy yourself the album. Watch out for excuses here ("I did limit my eating to mealtimes but I ate too many desserts so I don't deserve my reward). Many people are hesitant to treat themselves. Our culture encourages self-criticism and discourages legitimate self-reward. If you satisfied the agreement, you earned the reward. Remember, your reward may be a special purchase, some form of entertainment, or a personal treat; the most important criterion is that it be a pleasant and desirable experience. Buying yourself a pair of socks is not very rewarding if you would normally have bought them anyway! Finally, it should go without mention that your reward should not be fattening. The old pattern of food as a pick-me-up is one which you don't want to encourage.

Group members can be helpful to each other in the arrangement of contracts; if you do not form a group, we suggest you ask a friend or family member to be your witness.

4. *Procedures: Be specific.* Plan and clearly specify the mechanics of the group. Designate meeting time and place; one meeting per week is usually adequate. Some meetings should actually be eating situations—lunch or dinner, for example. This provides a laboratory for giving helpful feedback on eating patterns; it can also provide an occasion to experiment with lower calorie foods. Each member should have his or her own copy of this book. Development as a personal scientist must be basically a personal endeavor. The group is an aid, not an end in itself.

Finally, we suggest that you not admit latecomers; it is unfair to the group but much more unfair to the latecomer. Acquiring self-control skills, as you know, is a gradual, step-by-step process. It is essential to approach it that way—to begin at the beginning, not in the middle.

5. *Termination: Plan for weaning.* There *will* be a time in your life when weight won't be a daily obsession! You will outgrow your need for the group as such, though not for contacts with friends. You may find it helpful to phase out your meetings by planning them further and further apart. Or, you may want to continue meeting as friends; groups often strengthen friendships between members. If you plan to discontinue group meetings completely, you may want to agree that a member can call a meeting if a special problem arises. Whatever seems most helpful to *your* group is the option to pursue.

One final word. If your group is not working for you, and your efforts to improve the situation fail, do not hesitate to withdraw. Hopefully, you will have chosen members who are dedicated and trustworthy, and who will withdraw *only* if the group is not helpful and the chance for improvement looks slim.

ASSIGNMENT 2

Stage 1: Specify area. You are now going to practice your skills as an environmental engineer. You are going to try to assess and improve your social support system by applying some of the principles and suggestions you have learned.

Stage 2: Collect data. Your interaction with family and friends is an ongoing and complex phenomenon. For these reasons it can be difficult and unwieldy to record in very specific terms. Yet you do need to collect enough data on these interactions to allow you to tease out some patterns. We suggest that, for one week, you collect data on a 4 × 6 card for each day, using the format illustrated. In the "Person" column, list the individuals you have chosen to develop as support sources. The second column, "Their Actions," with its two categories, allows you to record two types of social behaviors which are important to your success. Rate each person's actions as *poor, neutral,* or *good* in each category; describe very briefly the actions which led to your rating. In the final column, "My Reactions," rate *your* reactions to each person's actions, using the same three categories (poor, neutral, fair). Write a short summary of your reactions, briefly noting improvements you could make. This format will enable you to individualize your engineering efforts, to assess patterns and trends in your interaction with each person. You can set aside 10 minutes or so each evening to review and rate your day. However, it is better if you keep your card with you during the day and record weight-related interactions as they occur. Two considerations should dominate here. First, you are trying to assess general patterns, not evaluate minute interactions. Second, recording should be simple and require a minimum of time. Record only enough to give you the general flavor of your social interactions regarding weight.

Person	Their Actions		My Reactions
	Helping Me Avoid Food	Feedback on My Efforts	
Kay	GOOD; she agreed to snack by herself.	NEUTRAL; she hasn't said anything.	POOR; maybe I'm expecting too much—I should have thanked her for snacking alone.
Dad	POOR; he still brings his beer and pretzels out at night.	POOR; teased me at supper about my new "fad diet."	POOR; at least he didn't offer me pretzels—I'll remember to thank him next time.
Aunt Mary	POOR; she brought over a cake tonight.	POOR; teased me about "wasting away to nothing."	GOOD; told her that her cakes are too good to resist. Asked her to help me by not bringing them over for a while.
John	GOOD; bought coconut cookies as a snack because he knows I don't like them.	GOOD; praised me for trying so hard.	GOOD; thanked him for his support; told him it helps a lot.

Social Support Log

Date _____

FIGURE 3

STOP! DO NOT READ ON UNTIL
YOU HAVE COMPLETED STAGE 2.

Stage 3: Identify patterns. By the end of a week some trends should be evident in your data. In your data analysis you should look for several things. First, who are the individuals who give you feedback—of any kind? You may find that some loved ones frequently make weight-related statements; others appear to be oblivious. Second, what kinds of feedback do various people give you? Does your spouse usually criticize, or praise? Do your children usually tease? Look for patterns in each person's interaction. Third, carefully examine your reactions. Do you respond in typical ways to certain types of comments, or to certain individuals? Are *your* reactions maintaining certain kinds of statements? Remember, social influence works both ways; look for *interaction patterns*.

Stage 4: Examine options. Now that you have a fairly clear picture of your social support system, or lack of it, what can you do to improve it? Review the guidelines for engineering; remember, *you* are the key person here. Try to tailor your plans to fit your loved ones. Your approach may differ, depending on the individuals you are dealing with. If your family is a close-knit one, with open communication, you might want to call a family conference to explain your efforts and your needs. If patterns in your loved ones' interactions differ greatly, it might be better to approach each person individually. For example, if you have a very supportive spouse, a very critical friend, and a very oblivious daughter, your approach with each may differ. Anticipate each person's reaction to your requests and needs. Some of your family members or friends may well be unwilling to help. In this case, an indirect approach may be best. Your only option may be to praise extensively *any* positive response on their part—no matter how insignificant. Others may be willing to cooperate to some extent. With these individuals, decide ahead of time what you need *most* from them. Is it too much to ask that they praise you initially? Is it enough to ask that they simply begin to decrease or eliminate teasing or criticism? Some loved ones may be generally supportive, only needing information from you about what they can do to help.

After your initial explanation (assuming there is one), how can you facilitate improvement? Can you give honest feedback on their efforts? Should you restrict your responses to praise for their efforts? How can you respond to teasing and criticism to reduce it—directly, or indirectly? Again, think in terms of individuals. In general, your most effective strategy is praise and positive feedback. In some cases, you may need to limit it to that. You may be able to give kind but honest feedback to some of your loved ones about what they need to improve; however, keep the emphasis here a positive one also.

Stage 5: Narrow and experiment. It may be helpful to make a list of the important persons in your social environment and your specific plans for enlisting their support. You might focus at first on your strong sources; discuss your plans with those individuals who are already generally supportive. Rely on support from these individuals while you develop other sources. For example, you might choose one person who will assume a very active role, who will warmly respond to whatever you request. You might choose another who is generally concerned but needs some polish. Finally, you might choose one person in whom you will simply begin to praise any interest shown in your progress, no matter how minute. If your family is already concerned and supportive, you can elicit assistance from all of them initially. If not, choose two or three individuals, and follow your tailormade plans for each. For two weeks, collect data, using the same form.

Stage 6: Compare data. At the end of two weeks, compare data. What patterns have changed? Have criticism and teasing decreased? Has praise increased? What about your reactions? Have you given enough positive feedback for their efforts? Have you responded to criticism with a gentle reminder or a sharp retort? You should be at least as concerned about your behavior as theirs—even more so. *Look for improvements;* remember, you're trying to establish a *positive* interaction system. Be aware, also, of individuals and patterns that have not changed. Reread the troubleshooting section. What can you do to change their behavior?

Stage 7: Extend, revise, or replace. What helpful changes can you make? Is it reasonable to ask certain individuals for more assistance? Or should you lower your standards somewhat? Watch your expectations. Remember that interaction patterns have long histories; they do not change overnight. The major criterion in social support is that *you* be satisfied with it. You may want to continue focusing on two or three individuals. If their support is insufficient, you will want to include others gradually. We suggest that you continue to collect data for a minimum of two more weeks, with more revisions then if necessary.

You should consider social engineering a long-term task, an ongoing project for the next few *months*. It is a long-term investment of effort, but one with a guaranteed long-term payoff.

8
Reducing with Reason:
The Personalized Diet

Since you are reading this book, you are probably a well-scarred veteran in the battle of the bulge. You may have gone on (and off) several dozen diets in the last few years and have surely read about many of the never-ending "miracle discoveries" which are reported in popular monthly magazines. When it comes to nutrition, you may already be well versed in calorie and gram counting. You have probably even memorized the number of calories in your favorite foods.

However, unless you are unusually well informed about nutrition, it is very likely that at least some of your opinions merit examination. For example, are you aware of the serious health hazards posed by some of the more popular diets? Did you know that some people have been hospitalized because of the nutritionally unsound diets recommended by best-selling books? Are you aware of the fact that most medical scientists do not agree with recent sensationalized reports of "miracle-working" hormones and "fat-metabolizing" drugs?

We will not spend time here discussing the potential dangers of the various reducing programs which seem endlessly to beguile the American public. New "miracles" are marketed each year and their popularity seems virtually unaffected by scientific reports on their dangers or general ineffectiveness. Those of you who are interested in a critical discussion of recently popular diets should consult the Consumers Union paperback *Rating the Diets*.

It would be all too easy at this point to give you a long and technical sermon on basic nutrition, digestive processes, and the physiology of fat metabolism. Besides putting you to sleep (or maybe making you hungry), such a sermon would probably not get across our major argument—namely, that *calories are not the only important consideration in dieting*. This overlooked fact has probably been responsible

91

for more weight reduction failures than any other. Calories are, of course, important, but they share the limelight with a number of other factors. For example, if your reduction program reduces caloric intake by eliminating any one of the three major food groups (fats, proteins, or carbohydrates), you are probably doomed to failure and you are risking some very serious health problems. You are in for similar trouble if you ignore the role of vitamins and minerals in your health.

Recall that the first step in personal science is to specify a general problem area. Are you sure that eating is a part of your weight problem? This may sound absurd, but the fact of the matter is that *not all overweight persons are overeaters!* That is, a person can eat a relatively normal amount of food and still have a weight problem. This is particularly the case with adolescent girls and some housewives. Is this a violation of the energy balance we talked about earlier? No; in fact, it is a vivid illustration of it. Research studies have shown that some obese persons actually eat fewer calories than some of their thin friends, but are so inactive that even their meager daily allotment of calories is greater than their caloric needs.

Even though it is likely that food consumption is a part of your weight problem, it is worth asking this question before you begin any personal experiments in dieting. At the end of this chapter we will indicate how you can go about answering the question. For the time being, let's assume that your personal data indicate that you are, in fact, eating too much. Should you immediately begin a diet? Not so fast! Even if you know that you overeat, you still need more information before you undertake a personal change experiment. There are at least three ways to overeat: (1) by consuming high calorie foods, (2) by eating *too many* low or moderate calorie foods, and (3) by doing both of the above. All three, of course, result in excess calories. We will refer to consumption of high calorie foods as *quality* control. Eating too much food will be termed *quantity* control. It has been our experience that most obese persons have both quality and quantity problems. However, *you* may be an exception to this generalization, which is why your personalized self-examination is so important.

What if you find out that you need to cut back on both high calorie foods and the sheer volume of your eating? Are you now ready to start a diet? Again, it is not as easy as all that.

To begin with, let's talk about the word "diet." The humorist Art Buchwald has suggested that the word *diet* comes from the verb *to die*, and many weight watchers would probably agree. If you have suffered through unsuccessful diets, you know that they may cause fatigue, hunger pangs, dizziness, and constipation. Altering your food intake does not have to be painful. As a matter of fact, it is our opinion that you should not begin or continue a diet that causes frequent discomfort. If it forces you to live with headaches or other side effects, it is probably not a nutritionally balanced plan. More important, if it is painful, you will be unlikely to continue it.

Another problem with popular dieting is that it encourages poor cognitive ecology. Going on a diet predicts that you will later go off it—and this usually means returning to the eating patterns that initially got you in trouble. Many diets encourage perfectionism by absolutely forbidding certain foods (NO butter, NO bread, NO fats, NO fun). As discussed in earlier chapters, these all-or-nothing laws force you to consider yourself a failure as soon as you eat one of the forbidden fruits. You have blown your diet and failed to be perfect. We therefore recommend that you avoid diets which are temporary or which *totally* prohibit a specific food category.

Because of its connotations, we would prefer not to use the term "diet." If you have been a weight watcher for some time, the very word may even make you shudder. It is unlikely, however, that many people will change their vocabulary on the sole basis of our recommendation. More important, the term "diet" is not itself the culprit. It is the hidden meanings ascribed to it that get you in trouble. When you hear the word, do you immediately think of painful semistarvation, or a temporary restrictive eating plan? These are some of the unfortunate associations which have prejudiced many weight watchers against the term. In what follows, we will use the word "diet" in the more general sense of a nutritional program. Be sure to keep this in mind as you read.

HOW TO EVALUATE A DIET

Let's assume that from past experience you already believe that you need to make some changes in your food intake. You now face two decisions: (1) what *kind* of diet do you want? and (2) how should you *implement* it?

This section will be devoted to deciding on the best diet program for *you*. In the next section we will offer some suggestions on how to be successful in adopting that program. Remember—in both of these areas, we will be talking about *general* considerations. The most important considerations for you, however, are *personal*—does the diet fit me? can I live with it? will it give me the results I want? The most important data in your weight control efforts are your own.

There seems to be an almost endless assortment of popular diet programs, ranging from the fat-free and carbohydrate-free to the high-protein and high-fat. Many popular magazines have their own favorite diets, which are often combinations of other eating programs. If you actually *believe* all that you read, you can't help but be confused by the array of diets which are marketed. One specialist tells you to eat carbohydrates but no fats. Another tells you just the opposite. Miraculous claims are made for the strategy of eating only one food—rice, yogurt, grapefruit, or fish. Some will tell you that alcohol and sweets can help you lose weight. Amid all of these sensational and often conflicting claims, how can you decide? Are there any guidelines that might assist you? We think so. In reading our recommendations, however, remember to allow some room for your individuality. If you have food allergies or are pregnant, for example, these are additional considerations that deserve attention.

1. *Your diet should encourage well-balanced nutrition.* That is, it should *not* totally eliminate any of the following food groups: meat (including fish), grains (including bread), dairy products (including eggs), fruit, or vegetables. This, of course, does not mean that a particular diet should not recommend discretion in how much you consume from each group. However, diets that prohibit foods of a particular category often risk nutritional imbalances that could be dangerous.

We promised to avoid a dry sermon on nutrition. Most of you may already be familiar with the concept of a balanced eating program—where approximately 25 percent of your calories are *protein,* 50 percent are *carbohydrate,* and 25 percent are *fat.* However, there are critical differences in the quality of various proteins, carbohydrates, and fats. This is part of the reason that we recommend that you eat something from each of the food groups. For example, there are some essential proteins which your body does not receive from most fruits, vegetables, or grain. Without meat or dairy products, you may run some serious health risks. Likewise, carbohydrate sources vary in their provision of other important substances (such as cellulose, vitamins, and so on). Obtaining most of your carbohydrate calories from processed sugars, for example, can be harmful. Finally, you are probably well aware of the importance of eating more polyunsaturated fats than saturated ones. Did you know, however, that some researchers believe that you may actually slow down your weight losses if you don't receive minimal amounts of fat?

So far, we haven't even mentioned the significance of vitamins and minerals. The sodium contained in table salt (and—if you own a water softener—even your drinking water) has been shown to influence the likelihood of heart disease. Likewise, vitamins have been shown to interact in complex ways with your metabolism, resistance to disease, and general well-being.

Have you read the last three paragraphs with an impatient "I already know that" attitude? Perhaps the crucial importance of balanced nutrition would be more compelling if we were to show you how some of your own previous dieting pains were due to poor nutrition. *How many of the following have you experienced while dieting?*

headaches
dizziness
fatigue
water retention
irritability
constipation or diarrhea
depression
skin disorders
indigestion or frequent hunger pangs

There is a good chance that poor nutrition was a contributing element. To repeat, if you adopt an imbalanced eating program, you increase the likelihood of (a) unnecessary personal discomforts, (b) a very short-lived diet, and (c) mild, moderate, or severe health risks.

2. *Your diet should allow you sufficient calories.* This may sound ludicrous, but some popular diets prescribe daily calorie levels that are much too low. Medical research has shown that crash starvation diets are very ineffective and often result in dangerous side effects (such as damage to muscles and vital organs). Your body cannot store protein or water-soluble vitamins, which means that they must be provided almost daily to prevent some serious physical disorders.

How many calories should you consume? That depends, of course, on your size, age, metabolism, and activity level. We can, however, offer some rough estimates. If you are a moderately active adult, each pound of bodyweight requires about 15 calories for its daily maintenance. Thus, to *maintain* a current weight of, say, 150 pounds you need about 2250 calories per day. Consuming fewer calories, of course, will result in weight loss. If your ultimate goal is to weigh 120 pounds, you can expect to "afford" about 1800 calories to maintain the thin you. Relatively inactive persons should allow only 13 calories per pound, and very active ones can usually afford up to 17 or 18 per pound. Notice, by the way, that you can increase your calorie allotment by increasing your daily activity levels.

Two issues merit discussion before we move on. First, your *rate* of weight loss can be roughly calculated by looking at the difference between your maintenance allotment and your daily intake. For example, suppose 2250 calories would maintain your current weight. If you cut back to 2000 calories per day, you create a 250 calorie deficit. Since a pound of bodyfat is approximately equal to 3500 calories, it will take you about 14 days to lose one pound ($250 \times 14 = 3500$). If you cut back by 500 calories per day (twice as much), it will take only 7 days (half as long) to lose that pound. And here is where weight watchers are tempted to cut back drastically in order to speed up their losses. Unfortunately, your physiology imposes some limitations on your rate of reducing. In general, if you are losing much more than 1 percent of your bodyweight per week, you are flirting with danger. Beyond that amount, an increasing part of your weight loss is probably due to water loss and destruction of "lean body mass" (muscles, organs, and connective tissue). We therefore recommend that you should not reduce any faster than 1 percent per week. As a màtter of fact, even this may be too fast in terms of developing permanently comfortable eating patterns.

The second point is that your total daily calories should never be less than 1200, regardless of your weight. Unless you are under a physician's care, adopting such a near-starvation diet can be very dangerous. It is almost impossible to attain balanced and adequate nutrition on so few calories.

3. *Your diet should encourage flexibility and choice.* If it offers only restrictive menus, don't even bother to start it. Instead, it should allow you daily flexibility in what and how much you eat. Diets which recommend "exchange systems" are usually easier to maintain than those which dictate approved meals. Likewise, if a diet absolutely prohibits any categories of food, it is probably less appropriate.

A sound diet allows you to accommodate exceptions. You can make room for vacation eating, special events (e.g., birthdays), and occasional treats by cutting back elsewhere. However, *don't abuse your freedom.* It is all too easy to make exceptions the rule. As many of you already know, the average dieter is an expert at excuses. Be honest with yourself and, more important, make sure that you always make up for the exceptions. The beauty of a flexible diet is that it avoids many guilt feelings and temptations to quit. On the other hand—like the permissive parent—it places greater emphasis on personal responsibility and rational choice.

4. *Your diet should not require radical changes in taste or lifestyle.* That is, it should not force you to eat unsavory foods or to totally abandon your old favorites. If it demands expensive foods, costly preparation, or special sacrifices, you are unlikely to continue it. As much as possible, your diet should encourage gradual and partial changes in your old eating habits. If you usually eat three meals a day, a new diet that requires two or six meals may be hard to put into practice. Incidentally, we recommend that you generally avoid programs that require fasts or meal skipping—these can actually jeopardize your progress. The omitted meal is usually breakfast or lunch. If you have tried this strategy yourself, you may have experienced its frequent by-product—namely, a late evening binge or an extra large feast at the next meal. The famished eater is often an overeater. That is, if you skip a meal you are likely to be extremely hungry by the time another meal is scheduled. Sitting down to a meal when you feel starved is often an invitation to disaster. Many people overeat when they break their fast. In fact, they often consume so many extra calories that they more than make up for the sacrificed meal. The net result is weight gain rather than weight loss.

5. *Finally, your diet should be potentially permanent.* Can you really *live* with it? This is an important question to ask when evaluating a diet. Are its calories reasonable? Does it allow you enough variety so that you don't feel hemmed in by prohibitions? Does it require unsavory foods or fasts? Do you dread starting it?

The importance of goal setting should be very apparent here. Most of us dislike radical changes in our everyday patterns. This is particularly true in the realm of eating. If a diet asks for sweeping alterations of longstanding tastes and habits, we are likely to find it irksome and pursue it only briefly. To be permanent, it must encourage very gradual and relative changes—which, of course, produce very gradual and relative weight losses. It is all too easy to be blinded by spectacular claims of short-term success. But, as we have repeatedly emphasized, the benefits of reasonable and gradual standards for change are reasonable and *permanent* success. It may be worth recalling here that the journey of a thousand miles begins with but a single step.

HOW TO IMPLEMENT A DIET

Once you have found or developed a suitable eating program, you will be faced with deciding how to put it into practice. This section is intended to offer some helpful suggestions in that regard.

1. *Develop a recording system for your diet.* This can vary tremendously depending on your preferences and the type of diet you have chosen. Although some people like to count their calories, this is not a necessary ritual in dieting. If you are using an exchange system (such as one of those listed in *Rating the Diets*) you need only count your daily exchanges, for example, two meat exchanges, three vegetable exchanges, and so on. One of the simplest systems is to rate yourself at the end of each day regarding your performance. A simple wall chart in the bathroom lets you tally your maintenance of the diet.

Initially, your recording system helps to quantify your progress. It focuses attention on those aspects of your eating which need some alteration. When you have settled into a more reasonable eating pattern, the recording system may become unnecessary. A few people continue it simply because of the structure and information it provides. Likewise, when you run into future episodes of slight weight gain, you can quickly re-introduce a record keeping system to help in your problem solving.

2. *Implement your diet gradually.* The most successful approach to self-change is usually one that relies on small, gradual steps. If you make drastic alterations in your eating habits, the new pattern will seem strange and you may become discouraged. Introduce the easiest changes first and gradually work up to the more drastic or comprehensive. For example, let's say that you have decided to (a) reduce your consumption of alcohol, (b) strive toward only two or three desserts per week, and (c) reduce your intake of bread. If (b) requires the least strain or change—that is, if it is the easiest option—then you should begin with it. After you feel *comfortable* with (b), then begin working on the next easiest change.

3. *Stack the environment in favor of your diet.* That is, engineer your world in such a way that it is easy to eat in accordance with your diet. This engineering, you may recall, can be physical, social, and private.

Physically, it is easier to stick to a diet when foods that are encouraged by the diet are more available than foods that are discouraged by it. For example, suppose you are trying to reduce your consumption of candy by substituting fruit. You can make your task much easier if you do not keep candy in the house. This may require some social engineering, however, if other family members want to have candy around. Can it be stored out of your reach or at least where it is least conspicuous? Will your family agree not to eat it in your presence?

Other aspects of physical engineering are also worth mentioning. First, if you are going to eat out, choose a restaurant that offers a wide variety of foods. This will enhance your chances of remaining consistent with your diet. Likewise, don't be afraid to order à la carte. If you have been invited to someone else's house, plan ahead. You can't dictate the menu there, so why not leave yourself some room for special foods by cutting back earlier in the day? Finally, it is usually a good idea to do your grocery shopping on a full stomach. There is some evidence that the hungry shopper tends to buy higher calorie foods. If you are not the grocery shopper in your family, you can at least voice your preferences on a list.

The social aspects of dieting are hard to summarize briefly. You usually do not want your diet to become the prime topic of conversation with family or friends. On the other hand, you *would* like their cooperation and support. The best way to obtain this is with a sincere and direct request. Remember, if you present your case in a joking manner, it will very likely be viewed as a joke. You need not be overly dramatic, but you do need to be earnest. Anticipate awkward situations in which a friend or relative stubbornly insists on your eating. Mentally rehearse how you can avoid or resolve that situation, and practice your solution mentally until you feel sufficiently prepared. Finally, and most important, remember to express your gratitude for the cooperation and thoughtfulness of family and friends. Just as their words of encouragement are often your most prized possessions, your words of sincere appreciation may make their day a much happier one. Let them share some of the responsibility for your progress and—above all—don't take their assistance for granted.

Private environments are critically important in weight control, as we saw in an earlier chapter. This is particularly apparent when you try to put a diet into practice. You must remain continually on your guard against the cognitive garbage that can pollute and destroy the best laid plans for reducing. Here are some frequent signs of poor cognitive ecology in dieting:

a.   impatience at rate of loss;
b.   extreme guilt or depression after deviations from the diet;
c.   obsessive thoughts about food;
d.   anxiety and fasting prior to weigh-ins;
e.   recurring excuses for dietary inconsistency;
f.   private monologues about the futility of the diet;
g.   frequent daydreaming about life after the diet has ended.

If any of the above strike a familiar note, you should pay special attention to your private environment as you implement your new diet. Use some of the techniques suggested earlier to evaluate and alter your thoughts and feelings about the diet.

4. *Commit yourself to continual dietary experimentation.* Even with the most reasonable and flexible of dietary programs you can expect to need some occasional changes. Your tastes will vary and you may go through phases in which you prefer different kinds of food. More important, there is some evidence that your food requirements decrease by 1 percent per year after age 25. This means that you will need to readjust your diet continually to meet your changing physiological needs. Therefore, when we talk about a "permanent" diet, we do not mean a rigid, unchanging program of eating. Rather, we are encouraging a commitment to permanent dietary adjustment, a preparedness for the change which seems to be such an integral part of life itself. Your skills as a personal scientist will prepare you to meet those changes with adaptive and precise counter-adjustments, giving you a maximally full and rich life. Don't hesitate to use those skills extensively.

ASSIGNMENT 3

You should now be ready for some personal experimentation. Be sure to devote at least four to six weeks to this assignment (preferably longer). Also, remember that its evaluation should depend on *behavior change,* not weight loss. Even with the best of diets and the most accurate of scales, your weight will hit one or more plateaus after the first two to three weeks of dieting. These "sticking points" are thought to be caused by periodic water retention following the mobilization (emptying) of fat cells. They usually recur at different intervals throughout a reduction program; the intervals probably depend on such factors as your rate of loss. However, the plateaus again emphasize the critical importance of using behavior change as the immediate index of improvement in your personal experiments.

Stage 1: Specify area. The general problem area here, of course, is food consumption. Remember that it is only part of the energy equation—we will discuss the other part (physical activity) in a later chapter. For the present assignment, you will be evaluating *what* you eat— the quality and quantity of your food intake.

Stage 2: Collect data. A frequent occurrence in your personal experiments will be the evaluation and revision of your record keeping system. You will usually begin with a rather broad and detailed system which allows you to identify patterns and evaluate the status of the problem. Later, when you have chosen a self-change strategy, you may want to condense your record keeping system to make it more relevant or manageable for the task at hand. This is particularly true with your diet experiment.

We recommend that you begin with a comprehensive system that will allow you to calculate your average daily intake of calories. This first self-monitoring system should also offer information on possible patterns (time of day, location, etc.) A form like the one below might be used:

Date _____		FOOD INTAKE RECORD			
Day of Week _____				Total Calories _____	
Time	Location	Food	Group	Quantity	Calories
8:15	Kitchen	poached eggs	dairy	3	240
	Kitchen	white toast	grain	2 slices	120
	Kitchen	butter (for toast)	dairy	2 pats	100
	Kitchen	milk	dairy	8 oz.	160
12:00	McDonald's	Big Mac Hamburger	meat, grain, & dairy (cheese)	1	600
	McDonald's	milkshake	dairy	8 oz.	320
.	.	.	.	.	.
.	.	.	.	.	.
.	.	.	.	.	.
.	.	.	.	.	.

FIGURE 4

Notice that each item in a meal gets a separate entry whenever possible. Also note the importance of having an accurate caloric guide, such as *The Brand Name Calorie Counter*.

The above system will require some effort on your part. Writing down everything you eat is not as easy as it may sound. It is important that you record your eating as soon as possible. Calorie calculations can be postponed until the end of the day.

STOP! DO NOT READ ON UNTIL YOU HAVE COMPLETED STAGE 2.

3. *Identify patterns.* After one week, you should have a relatively accurate sample of your daily eating habits. This presumes, of course, that your recording has been accurate and that you engaged in your typical eating habits during the week in question.

To analyze your personal data, begin by totaling each day's calories. Then calculate your *average calorie consumption* by adding together each day's totals and then dividing by the number of days. For example, suppose your data were as follows:

Wednesday	2740 calories
Thursday	2310 calories
Friday	2840 calories
Saturday	3150 calories
Sunday	2875 calories
Monday	2480 calories
Tuesday	2330 calories

Adding these amounts together gives a weekly total of 18,725. Dividing by 7, we find an average daily intake of 2675 calories.

Now then, your first question should be, "Am I consuming too many calories?" To decide this, we will resort to a little more arithmetic. Begin by rating yourself on the activity scale outlined below.

13	14	15	16	17
very inactive	slightly inactive	moderately active	relatively active	frequent strenuous activity

If you are a sedentary office worker or a housewife you should probably rate yourself a "13." If you supplement a sedentary lifestyle with occasional activities (such as cleaning, low exertion sports, etc.), circle "14." A score of "15" means that you frequently engage in activities which require moderate exertion (e.g., daily calisthenics, jogging, etc.). Most of you are probably "13s" or "14s." A "16" requires that you are almost always on the go, seldom sitting down or standing still for long periods of time. Do not give yourself a "17" unless you are a construction worker or otherwise required to expend considerable energy on frequent strenous tasks.

Recall that your activity rating gives an approximate calorie allowance for each pound you weigh. One way to decide whether you are overeating is to find your allowable calories for various desired weights. In the table below, find your activity rating and your desired weight for six months from now. (NOTE: your desired weight should not be less than 90 percent of your current weight—watch your standards!)

TABLE 5
Daily Calorie Allowances

Desired Weight	Activity Rating 13	14	15	16	17	Desired Weight	Activity Rating 13	14	15	16	17
90	1170	1260	1350	1440	1530	200	2600	2800	3000	3200	3400
100	1300	1400	1500	1600	1700	210	2730	2940	3150	3360	3570
110	1430	1540	1650	1760	1870	220	2860	3080	3300	3520	3740
120	1560	1680	1800	1920	2040	230	2990	3220	3450	3680	3910
130	1690	1820	1950	2080	2210	240	3120	3360	3600	3840	4080
140	1820	1960	2100	2240	2380	250	3250	3500	3750	4000	4250
150	1950	2100	2250	2400	2550	260	3380	3640	3900	4160	4420
160	2080	2240	2400	2560	2720	270	3510	3780	4050	4320	4590
170	2210	2380	2550	2720	2890	280	3640	3920	4200	4480	4760
180	2340	2520	2700	2880	3060	290	3770	4060	4350	4640	4930
190	2470	2660	2850	3040	3230	300	3900	4200	4500	4800	5100

Suppose your activity rating was 14 and your daily calorie average was 2675. The table shows that this level of food consumption will *maintain* a weight of slightly more than 190. Generally speaking, if your daily calorie consumption is greater than that allowed for your (six month) desirable weight, then you probably need to cut back on food intake.

Let's briefly consider the possible (but rare) person who finds that his daily calorie consumption is allowable—that is, that he is apparently not an overeater. Before drawing this conclusion, you should review several possible sources of error:

a. Is your activity rating too high? This is easy to overestimate. Would rating yourself as less active make your current calorie consumption excessive?

b. Were your food intake records inaccurate? This is also a very frequent error. Devote another week to recording everything you eat and be extra careful in your self-monitoring.

c. Are you now losing weight? This would indicate that you are, in fact, undersupplying your body and therefore mobilizing fat to make up the difference.

d. If all of the above fail to challenge your conclusion that you are not overeating, only two possibilities remain. Either (1) you are extremely inactive (e.g., a "12" or even a "10" might describe your activity level), or (2) you may be one of those very rare individuals who suffers from metabolic dysfunction.

Let's return to the rule rather than the exception—namely, most overweight persons are overeaters. What do you do after you have drawn this unsurprising conclusion? Your next search is for patterns. Are your excess calories contributed by excess volume (e.g., extra helpings), poor quality (i.e., high calorie "junk" foods), or both? What are the differences between at-home and away-from-home eating? Do you consume more calories on weekends or in the evening? Are any of the five major food groups (meats, dairy, grains, fruits, and vegetables) over- or under-represented?

4. *Examine options.* There are many ways to cut calories. Some of you might want to consider the formal diet plans which have been popularized over the last two decades. If so, remember to evaluate the diet on the criteria mentioned earlier. With the possible exception of a few of the exchange system diets, we are not very encouraged by the prospects of the popular diet programs. To be optimally useful for you, an eating program must be individualized to your tastes and habits as well as your caloric and nutritional needs. For this reason we usually recommend that weight watchers first attempt to develop a reasonable dietary program on their own.

One promising option involves substitutions. There are sufficient low calorie foods on today's market to allow you ample opportunities to cut calorie corners without too much trouble or expense. Look back at your food intake records. Where could the substitutions be used? How much would they save? You should try to overcome any initial prejudices you might have against lower calorie foods and substitutes. After a few weeks of taste adaptation, many people come to prefer the substitutes over their original food choices.

A third general option is to look for food items that could be reduced in volume. Remember, cutting back by only 100 calories a day will save you over ten pounds per year! Where could you trim your eating without too much sacrifice? Are dairy products over-represented? How about snacks? Again, look over your personal data and try to come up with comfortable ways of cutting back.

While you're doing that, it may be helpful to set a daily quota of calories to cut. We usually recommend that you multiply your current bodyweight by 2 and then reduce your daily calorie consumption by this amount. Cutting this amount of calories from your daily intake will result in a loss of about 10 percent of your bodyweight over six months. For faster and larger reductions, you can use 3 or 4 as the multiplier, but this often requires abrupt and extensive changes in your everyday eating patterns. We recommend that you avoid reducing your daily calorie intake by more than 4 times your current bodyweight.

5. *Narrow and experiment.* Select one or more specific strategies for reducing your daily food intake comfortably. Before you examine your strategy in a personal experiment, look back over our earlier suggestions on methods for implementing a diet. Next, decide whether you want to condense your record keeping system. If you continue monitoring all food intake, it will require considerable effort and attention. On the other hand, such a complete record will tell you whether your chosen strategy has produced favorable or unfavorable changes in other areas of your eating. If you choose to record only snacking, for example, you may overlook changes in regular meal consumption.

As a rule of thumb, we usually recommend that you condense your recording to cover only the foods that have been singled out for change. If, however, you suspect unfavorable changes in other areas of eating or you simply prefer the more complete recording system, don't hesitate to reinstitute it.

6. *Compare data.* Remember, your evaluation should rest on behavior change, not weight loss. Just before you evaluate your experimental results you may want to collect a few days' worth of total food intake. This will let you see whether (a) your total daily caloric consumption has changed, and (b) other aspects of your eating have been affected by your dietary changes.

7. *Extend, revise, or replace.* If your personal data suggest that your intake has been sufficiently reduced and you have not found your diet too demanding or dull, simply continue its practice. As long as it produces these satisfactory results, it remains a useful element in your reduction efforts. Over long periods of time, you may be tempted to discard your recording system (particularly if things are running smoothly). This is legitimate, but we recommend that you reintroduce self-monitoring (a) for a few days every month just to quantify your progress and possibly detect any problematical trends, and (b) at the first sign of difficulty.

Few diets are perfect, and this is particularly true of self-developed varieties. Usually, their imperfections lie in the fact that they either fail to trim enough calories or require too much in the way of personal sacrifice. Many people continually change their diets to insure variety and avoid the staleness of overfamiliarity. We view this continual dietary readjustment as a good habit since it keeps you well prepared for change and well apprised of your caloric intake. Don't hesitate to experiment with new food substitutions and different ways of cutting corners.

If your dietary experiment was relatively unsuccessful, don't jump to the conclusion that the inadequacy lies in *you*. Remember, in personal science, some of your self-change projects are bound to yield less positive results than you desire. Meeting these temporary setbacks with confident determination to try another solution is an essential part of the problem solving spirit. We are sincere in our insistence that occasional "failures" are very valuable experiences in your apprenticeship as a personal scientist. As you weather these occasional setbacks, you will develop a healthy resistance to the quick despair and "give-it-up" attitudes of so many unsuccessful dieters. More important, each of your negative outcomes provides valuable information about yourself. Are your failures often associated with inappropriate standards? Are your efforts usually brief? Had you begun them with less confidence or enthusiasm than other (more successful) experiments?

Finally, as you will soon discover, an initial setback is often followed by a successful second attempt. Your data from the first self-change project guide you in correcting your subsequent choice of solutions. We therefore suggest that you remember the apt comment of Francis Bacon, who said, "Truth comes out of error more easily than out of confusion."

9
Is Your Eating Style
a Problem?

Most dieters realize that *what* they eat can cost them calories; few, however, realize that *how* they eat may also be an important factor in successful reduction and maintenance. There have even been some recent suggestions by therapists that obese individuals should be given supervised courses in "remedial eating" to correct their aberrant habits!

You may be saying to yourself, "Come on, now—how many different ways are there to swallow?" Well, it turns out that there are quite a few factors that seem to affect the size and frequency of your swallows. That is to say, it is now believed that "eating style" may be a factor in how many food calories you consume. For example, do you tend to eat more crunchy and chewy foods than semisolids and liquids? How fast do you eat? Do you continue to eat as long as there is food on your plate? These and other factors have been suggested as having potential significance for your reduction efforts.

In this chapter we will explore a wide range of facts and theories about how your eating style can affect your weight. At the outset, however, you should be warned that scientific knowledge about the mechanisms involved is still very modest. We know quite a bit about the physiology of digestion and food absorption, but we know relatively little about the biological processes which are the basis for your sensations of hunger and satiety ("fullness" or satisfaction). The theories continue to be more plentiful than the facts, and the former are often in conflict. For example, several researchers have suggested that the *size* of your bites may make a difference. They disagree, however, on whether you should take large or small bites. A few theorists have even argued that there is an "obese eating style" that characterizes most overweight persons. In our opinion, the evidence is still much too meager to justify such a conclusion. The point of all this is to emphasize again the crucial importance of your personal experimentation. Theorists can argue all they want about what *should* work for *most* overweight individuals. The most important concern in your self-change efforts, however, is what *does* work for *you*. We will discuss the various factors that have been suggested as potentially influential. It will then be up to you to experiment and decide whether each factor is important in *your* reduction efforts. The assignment at the end of this chapter will give you specific suggestions on how to go about this.

THE EATING CYCLE

Including snacks and nibbling, the average individual probably eats almost 100,000 times in a lifetime. This may be a good figure to keep in mind the next time you feel guilt-ridden over a single unrestrained food orgy. *One* indiscreet meal, or even a binge-filled vacation, cannot undermine all of your other reduction efforts. It is the overall pattern which will tell the ultimate story.

One of the interesting questions in research on food regulation has dealt with the importance of meal *size* versus the *interval* between meals. What is the effect of eating a few large meals spread across the day rather than several smaller meals at shorter intervals? This question was initially suggested by the observation that animals tend to control their weight by altering the interval between meals rather than changing meal size. Could this strategy be successfully used by humans? There is some evidence that frequent smaller meals (e.g., four to six per day) may facilitate optimal conditions for food absorption and normal bodily functioning. This is particularly the case when specific gastrointestinal disorders are present. However, research to date has not found the use of frequent smaller meals very helpful in producing weight loss. Although a few individuals find it helpful, most do not. There must be other aspects of the eating pattern which are more critical.

What exactly is that pattern? Scientists interested in the physiology and psychology of eating have usually addressed their questions to one of three general areas:

1   the factors that initiate eating (What turns you on?);
2. the nature of the eating performance (How do you eat?);
3. the factors that terminate eating (What turns you off?)

Initiating factors have usually been lumped together into theories of hunger, while terminating influences are said to be relevant to satiety.

WHAT TURNS YOU ON?

Why do you start eating? Your first inclination, perhaps, is to say, "Because I'm hungry." Recent research evidence suggests, however, that we are frequently *not* physiologically hungry when we start eating. There is even some reason to believe that many of us are badly out of touch with our body chemistry when it comes to hunger. What we often call "hunger" may actually be anxiety and tension or boredom. We may be eating in response to emotional needs rather than our body's caloric requirements. This emotional form of eating will be discussed at more length in a later chapter. For the time being, suffice it to say that true physiological hunger is not always the cue for our eating. What are the other possible candidates?

Well, let's look at your various environments. In the private environment you have not only your physiology but also a variety of cognitive elements. *Thoughts about food are often followed by eating.* That is, you can make yourself feel psychologically hungry by thinking about eating. Most of you have probably experienced this in your previous diets. As food becomes a more frequent topic in your thoughts, it becomes more and more tempting to eat. Your life may eventually seem to be dominated by food, until you simply give up just to avoid continual persecution by your own thoughts. This may be another reason for the frequent failure of drastic calorie-counting diets—they force you to think about food so much that they may actually make dieting more problematical.

Another environment that may be important in eating is the physical world. Many individuals are unaware of the role of everyday physical cues in their feeding patterns. How often, for example, do you eat *because* of a clock? Many people find themselves eating at 8:00 a.m., 12 noon, and 6:00 p.m. regardless of their physiological hunger. It is so easy to adopt the eating patterns of our culture that you may end up relying on a clock to tell you when to eat! ("If it is 12 noon, I must be hungry!") Clocks, however, are not the only physical culprits that encourage you to start eating. Television commercials are another. Have you ever noticed how many tantalizing foods are advertised during prime time programs? You may have been comfortably watching a late evening talk show—totally content with your current physiology—when a commercial invites you to think about beer and pretzels . . . or mayonnaise . . . or corn chips.

But perhaps you were already aware of this fattening propaganda. That does not mean that you have been unaffected by it. This is often illustrated in your grocery buying. Even though you may hate commercials, you tend to buy name brand products that receive a lot of advertising. Most shoppers buy the brand that gets the greatest exposure in commercials and printed advertisements. But it is not just advertising that affects your buying and eating of groceries. Have you ever noticed how much emphasis your local grocer places on the sense of *sight?* Why are foods packaged in bright colors (especially red)? Why do they use see-through (cellophane) packages for candies and sweets? In the bakery section, why are cakes and pastries placed on decorative pedestals with delicate paper frills? Why are frozen foods usually packaged in a box adorned with a tantalizing picture of its contents? The answer to all of these, of course, is that they tend to increase sales. The grocer goes to great lengths to catch your eye (as well as your dollar). Have you even wondered why there are candy displays at the check-out counter? Think for a second—what do you do when you're waiting for the person in front of you to be checked out? Do you stand there with your eyes closed or stare at the floor? No, of course not. You look around you, and there they are—candies and cigarettes, day-old pastries and "Today's Specials." You are a captive audience while you're standing in the check-out line, and your grocer takes full advantage of that.

Some of you may now be feeling a little hostility toward your grocer for sneakily sabotaging your health, your diet, and your budget. Ironically, many of you are his guilty accomplices! Recall that seeing often leads to buying or eating. Do you often cue unnecessary eating at home by using some of the grocer's own tactics? Do you keep bowls of fruit, candy, or other snacks openly displayed in your house? When you open a refrigerator or cabinet door, what kinds of food stand out—tempting snacks? Do you keep serving bowls on the table when you eat meals? Each of these practices may encourage problem eating (as well as more frequent trips to your friendly neighborhood grocer).

Some researchers have suggested that there is an even more subtle form of diet sabotage than those discussed above. It presumably stems from the association of eating with various physical objects or locations. According to this theory, eating in a particular place can cause the development of food associations which will initiate future eating episodes. For example, if you frequently snack while sitting in your favorite chair, sitting in the chair may eventually come to suggest snacking. That is, the chair may become an initiating cue in and of itself. An entire room can also acquire these food associations. Some housewives report that just being in the kitchen makes them "hungry." The more places you eat, of course, the more likely it is that you will be frequently tempted to eat. If the kitchen, dining room, den, and bedroom are all associated with food, each one may come to initiate eating.

We have talked about private and physical cues which may turn on an eating episode. What about your social environment? Unless you usually eat alone, the eating habits and comments of other people can be tremendously influential in your own calorie consumption. How often do you start eating because someone else is eating? This pattern is particularly clear in late evening snacking and at parties. You may even be unaware of the influence. How many times have you decided you were hungry only *after* seeing someone else eating? A more pernicious form of social cueing, however, is the food offer. You're lying in bed watching the late show and your spouse says, "I'm going to make a sandwich—can I get you anything?" For many people, saying "No, thanks" in this situation is very difficult because it seems like an open rejection of an affectionate offer. This is also true in other social situations—when you are invited to just try something or are urged to have a second helping. In many of these predicaments, your physiology is content—you're not really hungry—and yet you accept the food offer to avoid seeming unsociable or rejecting. It is our opinion that many well-meaning spouses accidentally sabotage their partner's weight loss efforts by expressing their affection in calories. There are many less fattening and more satisfying alternatives.

So far we have examined some of the private, physical, and social factors which may encourage you to start eating. In this chapter's assignment, we will suggest ways of evaluating their role in your weight problem. Once you have started eating, however, there are additional considerations.

HOW DO YOU EAT?

We mentioned earlier that the way you eat may influence the amount you eat (calorically). The mechanisms of that influence are still unclear, but there is at least some evidence to suggest their potential relevance for your weight loss efforts. Scientific research on these issues has generally focused upon the nature of the food and the form of eating. These two factors are obviously related.

Now then, what do we mean by the nature of the food? This usually refers to characteristics of the food consumed. Among the factors which researchers have examined have been:

1. volume;
2. fat, protein, and calorie content;
3. mastication value (how much chewing is required);
4. tonicity (the food's concentration);
5. palatability (taste).

Each of these factors has been suggested as an important determinant of how much you eat. Unfortunately, their effects seem to be very complex and may vary from one meal to the next. More important, they may vary from one person to the next. Volume may be important in *your* eating but relatively less influential in the eating patterns of your spouse. The significance of personal experiments is once again apparent.

For some individuals, the sensation of fullness or satisfaction (satiety) seems to be related to the sheer volume of their food intake. Unless their stomach feels distended or enlarged, they may continue to eat. For a person like this, high calorie foods are disastrous since he may consume hundreds of concentrated calories in his pursuit of bulk. Low calorie, high bulk foods (such as some raw vegetables) may be helpful. Artificial bulk-producing drugs such as methylcellulose are generally ineffective due to their meager volume effects and their rapid exit (into the small intestines) when they are taken on an empty stomach. Some volume eaters find it helpful to consume large quantities of liquid before or during a meal. This practice is probably not very effective unless the meal itself is composed of predominantly liquid foods. The reasons for this will be more apparent after you have read about food tonicity (below).

Many theories about the physiology of hunger and satiety have emphasized the *kinds* of calories you consume. For example, the glucostatic theory suggests that you eat when your blood glucose (sugar) is low and that you stop eating when it is raised. Lipostatic theories emphasize a biological regulator which is sensitive to the fat (lipid) content of meals. Still other theories have defended protein values and temperature-sensitive mechanisms. The latter are illustrated in the fact that most people eat more when they are cold. To date, each of the various theories has had spotty success. There is evidence to suggest that each is at least partially true. For example, blood sugar levels do seem to influence some aspects of eating. The fat content of food also has been shown to affect your total food consumption. When your meal contains fats (lipids), a hormone (enterogastrone) is released which slows down stomach emptying, perhaps resulting in greater feelings of fullness. Likewise, high protein meals tend to stay in the stomach longer and increase your blood sugar and metabolism for several hours. The inclusion of both fat and protein in meals may therefore be helpful. High carbohydrate meals seem to present a variety of problems and seldom produce the enduring sensations of satiety which are helpful in avoiding between-meal snacking. If you eat a meal which is almost entirely carbohydrate (such as toast, a doughnut, or cereal and coffee), you may experience a brief "pick-me-up" sensation as your blood sugar is rapidly elevated. Unfortunately, some studies have suggested that this "cheap thrill" may be a very counterproductive one. Within 30 to 90 minutes your blood sugar will have returned to its former low level, sometimes actually falling *beneath* where you had started. If you eat in response to blood glucose, this is when you start feeling those intense food cravings. You may experience a sensation of dizziness along with such feelings as fatigue, emptiness, and a headache. For individuals who eat high carbohydrate breakfasts, this leads to that well-known episode of the midmorning munchies. You feel that you *have* to have something else to tide you over until lunch. If that "something else" is also carbohydrate (e.g., candy), the same vicious cycle is repeated. Moreover, if you consume excessive quantities of caffeine-containing beverages (coffee, cola), you may be adding insult to injury (particularly if you are drinking *both* sugar and caffeine). There is evidence to suggest that caffeine may reduce your blood sugar level, giving you the sensation of being hungry. Needless to say, supersweet coffee and sugary colas can be among the dieter's worst enemies. Interestingly, even though they do not seem to affect blood sugar, beverages which are sweetened by artificial means (e.g., saccharin) are often reported as producing a "pick-me-up" sensation without any adverse effects. In other words, you do not have to give up your desire for sweets in order to reduce— you can learn to satisfy it with nonfattening sweeteners.

It is worth mentioning here that the *sequence* in which you eat the various elements of your meal may also be used to your advantage. Again, since our research knowledge is still rudimentary, you are well advised to conduct some science of your own. Some general hints may, however, be helpful. First, it is important to realize that food leaves your stomach the same way it got in—one bite at a time. That is, your stomach empties into your small intestines in a gradual manner. When food enters the stomach and has been appropriately diluted and mixed, a small quantity is released into the duodenum. Like a miniature laboratory, the small intestine does a quick "lab analysis" of the nutrients and sends its report to the brain. If the food is high in protein, extremely concentrated (hypertonic), or high in fat, the brain will signal the stomach to slow down its emptying and may signal the rest of you to stop eating. If you are a rapid eater, of course, this important cue may be too late. Notice the possible implications of eating protein and fat (polyunsaturated, of course) early in the meal, and of eating more slowly. We will come back to eating pace and food concentration in a moment. For now, make a mental note of the potential importance of *what you eat when* in your meals.

How important is chewing (mastication) in your weight control? The answer is again far from simple. Some individuals seem to be able to regulate their calorie consumption better when they restrict themselves to liquid and semisolid foods. This is a difficult pattern to maintain, however, if you are trying to establish permanent habits. Other research has found that chewing may be a very important factor in how satisfied you feel after a meal. How often have you craved something crunchy or chewy? One recent study has suggested that normal weight individuals may tend to chew their food much more extensively than overweight persons. Could this be a factor in your satiety? A little personal science might provide the answer.

Food concentration, or tonicity, was mentioned earlier as a possible influence on your meal size. To be absorbed by your body, foods must be broken down into liquid solutions. When you consume a dry or solid food, your body must draw on some of its own stored liquids to dilute the food. These concentrated foods are called ''hypertonic'' because they create an imbalance or tension (tonicity) in your digestive chemistry due to their elevated (hyper) concentration. Salted peanuts and oatmeal are good examples. Have you ever noticed how thirsty they make you? This is because they have forced your body to give up some of its own liquids to digest them. Recent research has suggested that some individuals may eat less at a meal where the food is relatively hypertonic. However, if you are washing your meal down with extra liquid intake, you may be counteracting this influence. This may be one of the reasons that popular ''pre-loads'' (small snacks, liquid or solid, consumed a few minutes before a meal) are often unsuccessful. If, as some best sellers recommend, you drink large quantities of water (or diet soda) prior to a meal, you may actually be working *against* the helpful influence of food tonicity. Moreover, although it is a physiological myth that you actually ''shrink'' or ''stretch'' your stomach, it is a fact that your stomach tends to enlarge at the first sign of food. That is, your first few bites—or your pre-load—may make your stomach distend to prepare itself for further deliveries. We therefore urge caution and conscientious personal science in your flirtation with pre-loads. If they work for *you,* fine—by all means, use them. Be careful, however, that your pre-load doesn't cost you more (in calories) than you save at the meal. Generally speaking, the chances of pre-loads helping you reduce will be better if:

1. they are *very* low in calories (e.g., water, diet soda, raw vegetables);
2. they are very high in volume (e.g., two or three glasses of water);
3. they are the same general consistency as your upcoming meal (liquid pre-loads before liquid meals, solid pre-loads before solid meals).

Let your data be your guide.

The final food characteristic we will discuss is that of taste (palatability). Many popular diets recommend that you try to make your meals as tasty as possible—that you become a dieting gourmet. Unfortunately, your body makes this assignment a very difficult one. This is because:

1. you tend to eat more when foods taste better;
2. when you are dieting, your body becomes much more sensitive to food tastes.

One recent theory suggests that you are sensitive to food calories when your weight is stable, but that weight loss and dieting make you more sensitive to palatability. If this is true, the dieting gourmet needs to be very careful. Good-tasting dietetic meals are of little help if you end up eating so much that no calorie deficit is created.

In addition to the physical properties of the food you eat, the way you eat it may be important. It was mentioned earlier that increased mastication may help to regulate food intake. Another important factor may be your eating *pace*. Although it is still only preliminary, there is some recent evidence suggesting that rapid eating may lead to overconsumption. If you wolf your food down you may overshoot your biological needs. Moreover, some researchers have suggested that nutrient absorption and various aspects of your body chemistry may be impaired by eating too fast. Deciding whether you are a rapid eater may be difficult since our eating styles sometimes vary with different foods and social atmospheres. The following general patterns, however, are sometimes easily discriminated. Do you load your fork in readiness while you still have the previous bite in your mouth? How often do you put your sandwich or utensils *down* during a meal? Are you very quiet and preoccupied with eating when you first sit down? Do you often find yourself finished with your first helpings long before your eating companions?

We have now examined the potential importance of how you eat in calorie regulation. Did any of the factors sound close to home? Suggestions for evaluating their role in your eating style will be provided in the assignment. Meanwhile, however, we have only looked at part of the story. We have discussed factors which may encourage you to *start* eating and food characteristics which may affect whether you *continue*. But we have yet to discuss what makes you *stop*.

WHAT TURNS YOU OFF?

Assuming that you have started a meal or snack, what are the factors that encourage you to stop? As we examine these, the complex interrelationship among initiating, maintaining, and terminating influences will become apparent.

First of all, let's climb back inside your private world. Here, we may find some physiological cues which might signal you to stop eating. These, of course, are related to the food characteristics discussed in the last section. Perhaps the food is registering with your brain? If this is the case, it is often too late. Many people eat so quickly that they have far exceeded their body's needs before they hear that private quitting signal. This fact will provide one of the options suggested in your next assignment. For the time being, bear in mind that if you are, in fact, a rapid eater, your body chemistry is too slow to give you the best signal on when to stop.

It is possible (but perhaps unlikely) that you terminate your meal because of some private self-statement, such as "That's enough!" It has been our experience, however, that most overeaters end their feeding episodes because of one of three signals:

1. their physiological incapacity to hold more;
2. physical cues such as a clean plate, empty serving bowls, and so on;
3. social cues such as other people's finishing.

Do any of these sound incriminating? Perhaps some specific questions will be more helpful. How often do you feel "completely stuffed" after a meal? Is your plate usually clean when you finish eating? Do you sit at the table and nibble or take second helpings while you are waiting for others to finish? Do you feel guilty about throwing food away? If there are only a few bites remaining in a serving bowl or package, are you likely to eat them rather than save them? If you answered "yes" to many of these questions, it is likely that your terminating signals may be encouraging you to overeat.

We have now completed our discussion of the eating cycle. The number and complexity of possible influences may have surprised you. More baffling, perhaps, is how you should go about utilizing some of this new knowledge in your own reduction efforts. Let's have a look.

ASSIGNMENT 4

Stage 1: Specify area. The apparent complexity of eating style factors may make this particular assignment somewhat more challenging than the previous ones. You know that you want to examine your eating style, but how do you know which aspect to focus upon? That decision will have to await some personal data.

Stage 2: Collect data. To simplify your first glimpse at eating style, we suggest you use a form like the one illustrated below. It leaves out a few of the factors discussed in this chapter, but it may give you valuable tips on where to apply some more precise self-monitoring.

Begin by filling in the form each day for a full week. If your personal habits would be better suited by making some changes in the categories listed, by all means do so. Use your own judgment in deciding whether a particular factor was present. For example, you will have to estimate your eating speed and satiety. In general, don't mark a food thought unless you had been thinking about eating for several minutes beforehand. This is because most eating episodes are immediately preceded by at least one food thought.

STOP! DO NOT READ ON UNTIL YOU HAVE
COMPLETED STAGE 2.

Stage 3: Identify patterns. Now comes the fun part. After a week or more of self-monitoring, sit down and spread your data sheets in front of you. Tally the total number of times you checked each column. Also glance at your eating times and locations. Then try to answer the following questions.

Is your eating frequently influenced by the clock? This would be suggested by recurrent patterns in which you eat your meals or snacks at almost the same time every day.

Time	Location	Were you *thinking* about food beforehand?	Did you *see* any food before you decided to eat? (Include advertisements.)	Did you respond to a food offer?
8:15	kitchen	X		
12:30	Burger Chef			X
3:15	den	X		
6:00	dining room			(2nd X helping)
10:30	bedroom			

BEFORE

FIGURE 5

Are you being affected by too many eating locations? This pattern would be suggested by data showing that you eat in several different rooms while you are home (e.g., more than two).

What are the most prevalent factors in your eating style? Add up your total number of checks in each column. Those with the highest frequency of checks are probably in need of some personal engineering.

Stage 4: Examine options. Developing the ability to come up with effective problem solutions is an invaluable skill for the personal scientist. Some options may have begun to occur to you as you read this chapter. Before reading our suggestions, why not take a moment here to test your own developing skills. Write down as many options as you can think of for each of the prevalent factors in your eating style.

DURING				AFTER		COMMENTS
Did you consume a relatively large amount (*volume*) of food?	Did you *chew* it very little or not at all?	Was the food mostly *carbohydrate* (no fat or protein)?	Did you eat fairly *rapidly*?	Did you feel *stuffed*?	Did you leave a *clean plate* or empty carton?	
	X		X		X	breakfast (peanut butter on toast)
			X		X	lunch (fish sandwich and small juice)
					X	snack (cheese and crackers)
X				X	X	supper (rice casserole and salad)
					X	snack (apple)

If you are now reading on without having tried this brief self-examination, you may well be reducing your chances to develop independent self-control skills. It is often easier to rely on other people's suggestions or advice than to work on a problem solution by yourself. However, your ability to overcome future challenges in self-regulation may depend on the extent to which you practice and polish its component skills. The difference between successful and unsuccessful maintenance might be related to active versus passive participation in personal science. To the extent that you practice and expand the use of your problem solving skills, your chances of success are substantially increased. Don't just read about it—put it into practice.

Bear in mind that the option suggestions which follow are merely illustrations of some of the possibilities which you face. They are by no means exhaustive, and their usefulness for *you* can only be determined by *your* data.

If you found that your eating is often influenced by the clock, consider the various ways in which you could alter this pattern. How might you rely on your physiology rather than time to signal eating? Individuals who have fixed lunch hours because of their work can alter their breakfast so that they are in fact hungry when noon rolls around. Be careful not to skip entire meals if this leaves you starved at the next meal.

It should be noted that you can sometimes use the clock to your advantage in weight control. For example, if your snacking seems to be spread across the day without any obvious pattern, you can use a clock to impose some control. You might, for example, restrict yourself to snacking *only* during the first 15 minutes of each hour (1:00 to 1:15, 2:00 to 2:15, and so on). This does not, of course, solve the problem, but it introduces some degree of control. Later, you can stretch the interval between possible snack times (e.g., even hours only—2:00–2:15, 4:00–4:15) until snacking is within adequate limits. Notice that this use of the clock is intended to establish some control. When you work to avoid rigid time-bound eating patterns, you are trying to reduce control by the clock. Depending on your personal habits and the desired goal, either strategy may be worthwhile.

What if you eat in too many different places while you are at home? This pattern theoretically endangers your diet, since the more objects and places you associate with eating the more cues there are to signal future feedings. One option here is to restrict your eating to one physical location in the house. Don't just choose a room—choose a particular place in that room (e.g., sitting in *your* chair at the kitchen table). All eating (even late night snacks) should be done here. Some individuals also find it helpful to separate their eating from all other activities. That is, they refrain from reading, talking on the telephone, or watching television while they are eating. Don't snack while you are writing a letter, preparing meals, making up a grocery list, and so on. Otherwise, these various activities may come to signal eating by themselves. If you are watching the late show and decide you are going to snack, leave the television, go to your newly restricted eating area, have your snack, and then return to the television. This strategy not only weakens the control of your physical environment, it also reduces distractions that might prevent you from attending to other aspects of your eating style (pace, mastication, volume, and so on).

If food thoughts seem to be a frequent culprit in cueing inappropriate eating, you may want to review the Cognitive Ecology chapter. There are a variety of possible options here. One strategy which has been helpful for some people requires that you separate your food thoughts from eating. For example, if you have the sudden urge to eat, stop for a moment and do a mental replay of your last ten minutes' thoughts. Were you "obsessing" about food? If not, you may go ahead and eat. However, if you had been engrossed in food fantasies, set a timer for ten minutes and try to engage in some distracting activity. When the timer goes off, repeat your self-scrutiny. If you had not been obsessing about food, go ahead and eat (unless the urge has subsided). Otherwise, reset the timer. Be sure to adjust the time interval to fit your own patterns. If ten minutes never go by without a lot of food fantasies, reduce the interval to four or five minutes. Likewise, as you become more successful, lengthen the required separation between food thoughts and eating.

How about visual cues? Did you find that your urges often followed the sight of food? Let's look at some of the ways you might reduce this visual cueing. The more obvious options are to eliminate conspicuous food displays, such as bowls of fruit, cookie jars, and so on. Can you rearrange your refrigerator or cupboards so that snack foods do not catch your eye first? If the sight of other people snacking is a problem, can you request their cooperation in where they store or eat their snacks? If you frequently buy treats from a machine at work, are there ways to avoid the machine? Could you avoid carrying change? What are some other possibilities?

Food offers from others are usually handled best by a direct and sincere request—"I would really appreciate it if you wouldn't offer me food." If they forget at first, give them a gentle reminder. More important, make yourself a note to thank them every day or two until the new pattern has stabilized. If they catch themselves before completing a food offer, express your appreciation and comment on how helpful they are being. Let them know that their support and affection are appreciated much more when they are not hidden underneath a second helping or a late evening snack. If they buy or make you a favorite treat (candy, cake, etc.), thank them for the *thought* (not the gift). Do not feel compelled to eat it or compliment it—this will only communicate that you didn't really mean it when you asked them not to offer you food. The most important aspect of dealing successfully with food offers is to *watch for their absence!* It is easy to detect when a friend or relative has forgotten or refused your request. When people comply, however, it is easy for you to take them for granted. Take care to avoid this. Make a special effort to praise them—why not surprise them with a note or card conveying your appreciation?

Volume eating is often associated with feeling stuffed after a meal. There are at least three ways of dealing with this pattern. The first is to include a lot of high bulk, low calorie foods in your diet (e.g., raw vegetables, unbuttered popcorn, etc.). It is usually difficult, however, to include these in every meal. When they are absent, you will probably continue to overeat because of your reliance on volume signals to end your meal. A second option is to *introduce delays in your eating.* This strategy has been impressively effective with many of our clients. After finishing your first helpings, set a timer for 30 minutes and leave the table. When the timer rings, go ahead and eat another helping if you are still hungry. The amazing thing here is that most people feel completely satisfied after the 30 minute delay—their initial food intake has probably begun to take effect. It will take some effort on your part to execute this strategy, mainly because you will probably still *feel* hungry after your first servings. However, it is our opinion that this is one of the most powerful solutions for volume eating. Give it a try. After a while you will learn to stop eating while you are still mildly hungry—and you will feel triumphant when your body feels just as satisfied 30 minutes later on only half the calories!

The third solution for volume eating takes us into another category—rapid eating. Many people who eat too much also eat too fast. How might you slow down your eating pace? A long list of ingenious solutions has been suggested. It seems as though all of them have a critical common element—namely, they each make you more *aware* of your eating. For example, you can use unusual utensils (such as chopsticks) or eat with your nondominant hand. How about swallowing each bite before you put the next one on your fork? Some people actually put their utensils (or sandwich) down between bites. Since these are often dramatic changes from your old eating habits, it may be helpful to employ reminders when you begin. Put a bandage on your finger or wear some special cue on your hand. You may have to change cues to avoid getting accustomed to them. One of our clients even placed a small "slow down" sign next to his plate. Can you think of other possibilities?

This same type of cueing strategy can be helpful if you want to alter your chewing or the nature of your food (fat or protein content, tonicity, and so on). Some individuals have tried to count chews per bite but this turns out be a rather tedious and difficult task. The use of crunchy foods which require extensive mastication may be more beneficial. Also, remember that the usefulness of excessive liquids to distend your stomach or limit your food capacity may vary with the type of meal you are eating. Personal experimentation is again the most informative solution.

Did your personal data suggest that you eat for completion? Do you often leave a clean plate or finish off the remains of a food to prevent it from going to waste? When you eat at a restaurant, do you often force yourself to finish off everything you paid for? These are dangerous patterns. Remember that it only takes an extra 100 calories per day to put on ten pounds per year. If you consume the bits and pieces of leftovers as you clear the table, you are probably taking in at least that much. There are several ways of dealing with this problem. One of the more popular ones goes like this. At the beginning of the meal, place one bite of *each* food on the side of your plate and then work on what remains. When you finish eating, these three or four pieces of food should stay on the plate (to be thrown out). This strategy is designed to get you out of the habit of stopping only when your plate is clean. If you feel guilty about leaving food on your plate, that is a good sign that you are a completion eater. Beware of making excuses to avoid your assignment. Concern for ecology and unnecessary waste are commendable, but you are wasting a lot more if you jeopardize your health and happiness just to save a few pieces of food. Eventually, you won't have to waste the food. However, if you are a completion eater, it is wise to get over your hangup so that you won't be victimized in situations where you cannot easily control how much food is put in front of you (e.g., at restaurants and parties). As one dieter put it, it is better that the food go to *waste* than to *waist*.

Incidentally, if your self-monitoring data suggested that you sit at the table and nibble (or eat seconds) while waiting for others to finish, you have more options than just slowing your eating pace. For example, you *could* leave the table as soon as you finish. Many dieters dislike this solution because it may take them away from the family conversation and companionship of the supper table. A more popular option might be to take your plate and utensils to the sink (or dishwasher) and then return to the table. This reduces· the likelihood of seconds—but it may still allow you to nibble on foods. To solve this problem, one of our clients began knitting at the table while she talked with her family. By keeping her hands occupied, she made nibbling very unlikely. This solution is noteworthy since it illustrates the role of initiative and creativity in personal science. Don't be afraid to brainstorm for possible solutions. Our ingenious client, incidentally, has maintained a loss of nearly 50 pounds over two years.

Stage 5: Narrow and experiment. The most important thing to guard against in the present assignment is ambition. We have discussed a large number of possible problems and a variety of potential solutions. If you try to implement too much too soon you may undermine your own success. We suggest that you choose no more than *three options* related to your most prevalent eating style problems. Continue your personal data collection by using the previous recording form or a modified version. We recommend that you devote a minimum of two to four weeks to evaluating these options. Remember to use some mental practice in anticipating problems which might develop with your selected options.

Stage 6: Compare data. Have you encountered any difficulties in putting your problem solutions into practice? Do your personal data records suggest improvement, no change, or increased difficulties? How do they compare with your prior data?

Stage 7: Extend, revise, or replace. By now you should be able to spot some of the factors that may undermine an experiment. Did you set your standards too high? How accurate were your data? Were you conscientious in implementing your solutions? How might you have improved your chances of success?

If your personal experiment resulted in some improvements in your eating style, consider ways of continuing or expanding your strategies. Can you introduce some new or revised options to produce further changes? Remember that your eating style is the product of many years' experience. You are not going to renovate it overnight. We suggest that you curb your eagerness to move on to the next chapter until you feel comfortable with your revised eating style.

10
You Don't Have to Be Radical to Be an Activist

Congratulations! At this point you are well on your way to becoming a seasoned personal scientist, an *effective* campaigner in your personal war against weight. You are probably a better informed consumer—getting greater nutritional values for fewer calories. Your cognitive ecology is improving; you are talking to yourself about your weight control efforts in more reasonable and appropriate ways. You are learning, through well-planned practice, to approach each weight-relevant problem area as a personal scientist. In short, you are developing useful and permanent self-control skills that are applicable not only to weight control, but to other aspects of your life as well. Your self-statements at this point should be generally positive (though not perfect) and your monologues should be encouraging. You are well-deserving of frequent and genuine self-praise.

With some successes as a personal scientist under your possibly looser belt, you are ready to attack an area that has seen more lost battles—and more deserters—than perhaps any other in weight control: that of *exercise*. Few weight-relevant topics are as replete with fallacies—or failures—as this one.

What is *your* status as an activist? Your reaction to that word may quickly tell you. Does the word "exercise" elicit images of boring and tiring calisthenics? Does it remind you of those gadgets—sauna belts, cycles, weights, and the like—that are collecting dust in the basement? Does it cue memories of all those exercise programs you've started only to drop after four or five days, when exhilaration was replaced by exhaustion? If sit-ups and sweatsuits are your associations with exercising, your exercise history is probably characterized by failures. You are probably a staunch believer in several false assumptions about the role of exercise in weight control.

Many people who are well read in nutrition are surprised to find that they are virtually illiterate when it comes to the facts about exercise. You may well be one of those individuals. The importance of exercise as a critical variable in weight control has been underemphasized, misunderstood, even blatantly ignored—not only by the public but by many of the originators of the popular diets. And, unfortunately, this misunderstanding has profound consequences for weight control. *If you are not an activist, you are forfeiting half the battle in weight control.* You're not even fighting it. If you do not have and are not using the facts about exercise, you are missing half your opportunities for successful and comfortable weight control. You are working at half capacity toward becoming a slimmer, healthier you.

Stop and think for a moment. You have learned that in weight control, energy balance is the critical factor. Your weight is a function of the balance between your intake and your output of calories. Though several factors may influence it, that balance itself reigns supreme. If your caloric intake exceeds your caloric output, you will gain weight. If the opposite is true, you will lose weight. If the two are equal, you will maintain your current weight. The energy equation says two things: calories *do* count, and so does exercise.

Did you know that increasing your activity level will result in *greater and faster* weight loss—and a higher probability of maintaining your desired weight after you've reached it? Did you know that expanding your exercise patterns can *decrease* your appetite? Are you familiar with the beneficial effects of activity on good health and lowered risk of cardiovascular disease? Are you aware of the indirect impact of increased activity on improving nutrition? The facts are: exercise does all of these things, and more.

Now, you may be wondering—if these are the facts, why is exercise so underrated as a factor in weight control? If so, good for you. Skepticism is a healthy scientific attitude. The discrepancy between the facts and the fallacies in the role of exercise is rather puzzling at first glance. It is certainly legitimate to ask what has created this discrepancy. What factors have contributed to our collective failure to take advantage of the benefits of exercise—benefits for weight control, health, and general happiness?

"Obesity is in many instances clearly 'a disease of civilization.' " Many weight control experts concur with this statement by Jean Mayer; obese individuals are often victims of modernization. Reduced activity resulting from the mechanization of our world is possibly the major factor in the increased incidence of obesity in our culture. Modernization has decreased our activity level; it has simultaneously increased the availability of a variety of foods. A quick trip down the aisle of a supermarket documents the effect of modern methods of food preparation and preservation on our diets; we literally have at our fingertips hundreds of foods that are easy to prepare—and frequently loaded with calories. Yet, in spite of convenience foods, the evidence indicates that *we eat less, and consume fewer calories, than our grandparents did!* Your own experience may suggest that very fact. Many of you may have fond memories of Grandma's dinner table, loaded with a *variety* of hot breads and desserts, rich gravies, and greasy meats. You may also remember, however, the amount of work that was necessary to get that meal on the table. In most cases, Grandma had raised, preserved, and prepared the vegetables herself. She had baked the breads and dessert herself. And after dinner, she washed the dishes and the table linens herself. Grandma could afford to eat more, because she spent more calories.

Let's translate this state of affairs into energy equation terms. Generally speaking, our intake of calories has decreased slightly in recent decades. But our output of calories has declined drastically. In other words, intake is proportionately greater than output. The result is a positive energy crisis; an increasing number of individuals are spending fewer calories than they consume, even though they are consuming less than their ancestors did. Exactly what does this mean? If you are obese, your problem may not be that you are overeating. In our culture particularly, it may be that you are underspending.

In energy equation (input-output) terms, our culture is literally killing us with "conveniences." We live in a push-button world in which step saving is the goal. Look at the effects of mechanization on transportation. Why walk when you can ride? For many individuals in our culture, walking is almost obsolete. We spend our money driving around parking lots looking for the space nearest the store. We spend our time waiting for elevators to transport us from one floor to the next. Stair climbing burns up more calories per minute than practically any other activity; in our country it is virtually a lost art! It is difficult to watch television for more than a few minutes without seeing something advertised that will save us hundreds of steps. Unfortunately, these same "conveniences" will collectively cost us hundreds of pounds per year. Extension telephones alone "save" several miles of walking per year; their effect on collective poundage over a five-year period is staggering. Stop and seriously consider the number of "work-savers" that you have in your home or office, many of which you use every day. Can openers, dishwashers, garbage compactors, knife sharpeners, electric tools, lawn mowers—the list goes on and on. Even tooth brushing has become a power-operated endeavor!

Unquestionably, mechanization has drastically affected the workload of the average individual; it has also affected his entertainment. Our favorite form of entertainment seems to be sitting—sitting and watching someone else do something. Again, the list of examples is lengthy. Television is probably *the* prime example. Think how many hours per year people spend sitting, watching—and eating. That total would stagger the imagination. It is interesting to note how often spectator forms of entertainment are associated with eating. Snacking in front of the television is a familiar phenomenon. At many sports events food is actually hawked in the aisles; it is unnecessary to expend calories even to obtain it.

In considering our generally decreased activity level and its problematical effects on weight control, one point deserves clarification. Most people in our culture do not perceive themselves as sedentary—even when, calorically, they are. It is very easy to confuse being *busy,* or being *tired,* with being active. Unfortunately, a busy, even hectic, schedule—and fatigue at the end of the day—do not necessarily reflect calorie expenditure. You may very well be just as busy, and just as fatigued, as Grandpa, but for different reasons—reasons that do not involve high caloric output. As we have seen, the *nature* of our work has changed. A housewife's hectic day or an office worker's busy schedule may be every bit as "tiring" as our grandparents' days, but the difference in calorie spending is significant. It is important to note that tasks requiring mental concentration result in a type of fatigue—but in *very* minimal calorie expenditure (usually between one and two calories per minute).

Few individuals would be willing to return to Grandma's world; the benefits of modernization need hardly be elaborated. Modern science has improved our health, lightened our workload, and made possible many opportunities that contribute immeasurably to health and happiness. Yet, in many cases, the emphasis on step and time saving has become extreme, and the price we've paid has been high. Too frequently this emphasis has decreased activity level to the danger point in the energy equation—the point at which excess weight is maintained and additional weight is gained.

Modernization has had its influence, but another factor has also played a major role in the de-emphasis of exercise in our culture. That factor is the set of myths that continue to be perpetuated about the futility of exercise as a weight control strategy. We will consider two primary ones. The first myth argues that exercise does not burn up enough calories to be "worth it"; it says that the role of exercise in calorie expenditure is insignificant. This is the old belief that it takes several hundred push-ups to burn up the calories in a doughnut. It is the assumption of Herculean efforts for small returns. The second myth is that exercise always increases appetite. Why exercise more if it means you're going to eat more?

Your faith in these two fallacies may be encouraging you to work on only half the energy equation. If so, you are working on only half the problem in weight control. Step saving needs to be discarded in some areas; you need to become a caloric spendthrift.

FACTS AND FALLACIES: THE ADVANTAGES OF ACTIVITY

The first step in personal science is to get the facts. Let's check out some of the data on the effects of activity, or exercise, on weight loss, weight maintenance, and general physical fitness.

Exercise and Weight Loss

1. *Exercise is the critical variable in energy (calorie) expenditure.* As we have stated above, activity level is the major factor in the output half of the energy equation. Contrary to popular opinion, it is the *key* to calorie burning.

The human body requires (uses) energy for at least three major functions. The first of these is the maintenance of vital functions—

respiration, heartbeat, regulation of body temperature, and many other activities which your body performs automatically. Energy used by these functions is referred to as "basal energy." Your body uses energy at a particular rate to maintain your vital functions; this rate is your basal metabolic rate.

In addition to the energy required for basic maintenance, the body uses a small amount of energy in metabolizing food. Energy expended in this way represents a rather small percentage of the total energy requirement (expenditure). As we have seen in an earlier chapter, basal metabolic rate varies from person to person; most studies, however, show no significant differences in metabolic rate in obese and nonobese individuals. Nor does the expenditure of energy in food utilization differ in obese and nonobese persons.

The third factor in the body's total energy expenditure is that of exercise, or physical activity. Energy is expended in supporting and moving the body. It is this factor that is the *critical* variable in energy expenditure. Unlike the other factors in energy expenditure, exercise often differentiates the obese from the nonobese individual.

This difference in energy expenditure through exercise *may* begin as early as infancy. Some research has shown that obesity in infants as young as four months old was correlated with inactivity—but *not* with excessive food intake. This same pattern has been found in both adolescents and adults. Some studies have shown that obese adolescent girls actually ate less than their nonobese peers—but their activity level was *much* lower than that of their slimmer friends. It has also been demonstrated (via movies) that during the same exercise periods, obese girls spent much less time moving than did the nonobese girls. Similar patterns have been found with adults.

These data strongly suggest that the critical variable in energy expenditure is activity. They also indicate that obese individuals often miss their greatest opportunity to increase caloric output. Ironically, they are missing an even greater opportunity than their thinner cohorts. The obese individual actually burns *more* calories than the nonobese person when performing the same activity. The person who is overweight burns up more calories doing the same amount of work! He is therefore forfeiting an even greater chance to increase his output and to lower his weight.

2. *Exercise in moderation may actually decrease appetite.* If this surprises you, you may not be aware of the intricate workings of your body in maintaining a balance between your intake and your output, that is, in regulating your energy balance. The physiological mechanisms that govern the energy equation function best when *normal* ranges of activity or exercise are present. Let's be more specific. The body is "tuned" so that activity level affects appetite. When you are moderately active, your body is very efficient in regulating appetite and food intake to match your calorie expenditures. If you are inactive or sedentary, however, this efficiency is lost and you usually consume more food than you need. Therefore, contrary to the popular myth, moderate exercise may actually *reduce* (rather than increase) your hunger and food intake. Note the dual advantages of physical activity. Not only does it spend calories, but it helps to tune your hunger-controlling mechanisms. If your activity level is not in the normal range, your body is probably not functioning properly in regulating your energy balance.

3. *Moderate exercise combined with moderate caloric restriction is the most effective method of weight control.* Let's stop and review for a moment. Your weight is a function of the energy equation—the relationship between caloric intake and output. To lose weight, output must exceed intake. The data we have just reviewed on the effects of exercise strongly support its role in that equation, for they suggest that it affects both sides. As we have seen, exercise is the major variable in caloric output. It also influences caloric intake through its effects on appetite.

Does this mean you can forget about caloric restriction, as long as you exercise? No, it does not. Your best bet is to work on both aspects in moderation. In fact, you are in trouble if you work on either aspect to the exclusion of the other. In either case you quickly reach a point of diminishing returns. Severe caloric expenditure results in weight loss, but also in nutritional deficits and "cognitive claustrophobia." *Excessive* exercise results in weight loss, but also in serious risks to health and fitness.

We have already seen that *moderate* exercise may decrease your appetite. It is interesting to note that the benefits of moderation do not end here. The helpful effect of moderate exercise seems to be greatest when caloric restriction is also moderate. It becomes *decreasingly* effective when combined with excessive caloric restriction, possibly because of metabolic compensation for the restriction.

There are further benefits in a combination of moderate diet and exercise. This combination seems to increase the rate of weight loss as well as the amount—and to result in fewer effects (such as fluid retention) during loss.

If you have not appreciated your body as an intricate and finely tuned instrument, we hope you are beginning to do so. Fad diets which de-emphasize or ignore exercise—and which "push" one category of nutrients—become very questionable as one gains appreciation for the body's balances. The human body operates most efficiently when its delicate physiological balances are understood and protected.

Exercise and Weight Maintenance

Exercise is a crucial factor in weight maintenance as well as in weight loss. This should come as no surprise following the realization of its role in the energy equation. As we have seen, regular exercise allows room for and even works best with moderate caloric restriction. We have already noted that moderate restriction of food intake, instead of drastic measures, allows greater variety and better nutrition in your diet, as well as better cognitive ecology. The active individual is, therefore, more likely to maintain his desired weight once he has reached it. Exercise is beneficial in another way in weight maintenance; it provides, in Mayer's terms, an "automatic self-correcting mechanism." In the physically active person any increase in calorie intake *above* the energy balance level will result in minimal weight gain because the activist will spend more calories in moving his excess pounds. The sedentary person lacks this insulator against weight gain. He will spend fewer calories than the activist in moving his excess weight—simply because he moves less. Consequently, he tends to gain weight more easily and more quickly than his more active peer. Activity produces benefits, not only in weight loss, but in long-term maintenance as well.

Exercise and Health

Exercise is important not only in weight control, but also in health and general physical fitness. In addition to improving muscle tone and facilitating circulation and digestion, it is a preventive factor in cardiovascular diseases. Regular exercise reduces cardiovascular stress, lowers various serum lipid (fat) levels in the blood, and helps alleviate high blood pressure.

If you are an activist, you are decreasing your chances of a heart attack and increasing your chances of enjoying general good health. Further, as a spouse, a parent, and a friend, you are helping your family and your friends to do the same. Activity patterns are, for the most part, learned. Children imitate activity patterns, just as they do eating patterns, and activity level seems to be a factor in weight control even in infancy. Throughout childhood and adolescence it is critically important. In an earlier chapter we discussed the theory that childhood obesity involves an increase in the number of fat cells, which may make weight control more difficult throughout life. Whatever the reason, weight control in adulthood appears to be easier following a slender childhood and a fat-free adolescence. Your *active* life may be beneficial, not only to yourself, but to others around you.

When the beneficial effects of exercise are considered, the importance of increased activity in successful weight control becomes quickly obvious. We again suggest that you check the data for yourself; it is only when myths are replaced by facts that your exercise cognitive ecology will begin to improve. Your monologues and your goals concerning exercise may need as much revision and improvement as your exercise habits themselves. As we review some guidelines for establishing effective and permanent activity patterns, and as you implement your individual changes, remember to check your cognitive ecology frequently. *Don't stop using your head while you concentrate on using the rest of you!*

Remember, you may well be a victim of both the myths about exercise *and* modernization, or step saving. Watch your monologues and thoughts about exercise; make sure they are factual and realistic. Your thoughts about step saving will need special consideration; you may be surprised at the extent to which calorie saving has been your goal. Are you irritated when the elevator isn't working? Do you complain when you miss your bus and have to walk the seven blocks to work? If so, your attitude is probably one of calorie saving; it must be replaced by one of calorie spending. Our culture, as you know, will frequently remind you of the former. Therefore, you will need to assume a very active role in cleaning up your cognitive ecology in this important area.

EXERCISE ECONOMY: GETTING THE MOST FOR WHAT YOU SPEND

Several general guidelines may help you change your exercise habits in effective, permanent, and healthy ways.

1. *Exercise equals increased activity, not calisthenics.* This first, crucial guideline is a restatement of a major theme in successful weight control: if you can't live with it, don't start it. Above all, your exercise habits must be comfortable. If they are not, you will not continue them. The problem with going on an unreasonable exercise program, as with going on a restrictive diet, is that at some point you will probably go off it. Physical activity should not be a brief project; it should be a way of life.

The most effective and permanent way to increase your activity level is to develop an active daily routine you can live with. This can be done by making simple changes in your *current* daily activities. In other words, do what you usually do, but do it in a way that expends more calories. Stop and consider the variables that make this approach so effective. First, as we have noted, your major concern is *permanent* weight control. Moderation—and reasonable comfort—in all your weight control endeavors is your best guarantee of being slender—and staying slender. For most individuals, the most comfortable way to become, and to remain, an activist is to make adjustments in their current routines.

This approach has additional advantages as well. For example, it is portable. You are going to be performing routine daily tasks for the rest of your life—wherever you live. Adjusting your daily activities for greater caloric expenditure is not a seasonal event, and it requires no special equipment.

Is this approach *effective?* A good question—and one which you could probably answer fairly accurately at this point. You have already learned that exercise has a beneficial effect on both sides of the energy equation. It greatly facilitates caloric expenditure. Further, regular and moderate exercise may decrease appetite, and intake—when it is regular and moderate. Incorporating greater calorie spending into your daily routine provides possibly your very best opportunity for regular and moderate exercise habits.

Now, what kinds of changes are we talking about? Specific examples are plentiful. The first step is to establish that habit of asking yourself, "How can I spend more calories in performing this task?" You can answer the extension phone farthest away from you, instead of the nearest. You can look for the parking space farthest from the store. You can avoid elevators, and search for stairways. *You* can carry out your groceries. You can stand instead of sit, you can walk instead of ride. The list goes on and on. Your day is literally filled with activities that you do the easiest way. You will be amazed at the number of steps you save per day—steps that could be burning up calories.

Let's qualify an important point. We are not recommending that you exclude more vigorous types of exercise from your life—if you *enjoy* them. There are benefits from more strenuous exercise. Swimming, tennis, cycling—these are but a few of many activities that pay good returns in health and fitness. If you already enjoy, or can learn to enjoy, a more strenuous activity, that's great. You should pursue it.

We are saying, however, that it is a myth that activity has to be radical to be effective. *You do not have to sweat to be slender.* The idea that exercise must be strenuous to be effective is a harmful notion that sabotages far too many activist efforts. Concentrate on regular, moderate exercise through *increased,* not exhausting, activity.

2. Increase your activity level in ways that maximize caloric expenditure. In other words, get the most for your exercise money. You do not have to become an expert in physiology or body mechanics to accomplish this task. However, a few general principles may be helpful in optimally increasing your activity levels. First, activities that use large amounts of muscle mass burn more calories than those utilizing small amounts. Activities involving *all or large portions of your body* optimally increase calorie expenditure. You will, for example, burn more calories using your arm muscles than your finger muscles. The greater the muscle mass involved, the greater the energy (calories) expended. Activity involving your leg muscles is especially good; the muscle mass concentration in your legs is one of the largest in your body. Obviously, activity involving most or all of your body muscles is most beneficial.

Second, activity that involves moving your body through space burns more calories than more stationary activity. In other words, moving your body a given distance will generally burn more calories than stationary movements. Transporting your body two miles will burn more calories than transporting it one mile. The greater the distance you cover, the greater the calorie expenditure.

Third, the critical factor in energy expenditure is the *amount* of work done, not how vigorously it's done. This principle may surprise you, so consider it carefully. It is related to the one we just discussed—moving your body through space. *Covering the same distance generally burns about the same number of calories—no matter how it's done.* That's right. In terms of calorie expenditure, running, jogging, and walking briskly burn about the same number of calories per mile! Running a mile as opposed to walking a mile may save you time, but it won't necessarily burn up more calories. That's why it is a myth that exercise, to be effective in calorie expenditure, has to be exhausting, or even vigorous. In terms of calories burned, the main advantage in running a mile instead of walking it is that you can cover it more quickly—and maybe have time to cover a second mile. Remember, you burn calories by moving your body, by covering distances.

Notice that we have been talking in terms of calorie expenditure only. There *are* some benefits to be gained from vigorous exercise, however. It is vigorous activity which asks your heart and lungs to do more work—which is why breathing and pulse increase when you're performing it. These results of more strenuous activity have the beneficial effects on your heart and your cardiovascular system mentioned earlier in our discussion of exercise and health. A word of caution is in order here. It is advisable for individuals with cardiovascular problems to engage in activities that increase pulse and respiration *no more* than the increase resulting from light exercise. These benefits from vigorous exercise are important ones for your health. That is why we suggest you pursue an enjoyable, more strenuous activity in addition to increasing your daily activity load.

Finally, activity that involves moving your body vertically burns more calories than activity involving horizontal movement. The reason is simple: *gravity*. Vertical activity involves movement of your body against gravity, which increases the number of calories you burn.

Climbing stairs burns more calories than almost any other activity—
more than swimming, running, etc. One activity that equals it in calorie expenditure is walking uphill on skis on hard-packed snow! Any
activity that involves climbing is excellent for calorie expenditure.
You have a prime opportunity to burn calories if your home or your
office building has a stairway. Stair climbing is usually available and
it's cheap! It's an excellent strategy to include in your daily routine.

   3. Start off slowly. The third guideline is simple, but important.
Even increasing your daily activity level should be done gradually.
More strenuous exercise habits should be developed slowly and cautiously. Increases that result in excessive fatigue or in muscle soreness
will not be helpful if you are too tired, sore, or frustrated to continue
them. Individuals with known cardiovascular problems should be
especially cautious in this regard.

   **4. Program your environments to assist you in becoming an ac-
tivist.** Notice that "environments" is plural; your cognitive, physical,
and social environments may *all* need rearranging.

   We have already discussed the importance of actively revising
your attitudes toward calorie spending. The content of your thoughts
about increased activity should be data-based. Your goals for becoming an activist should be reasonable and comfortable. Your
self-statements should be realistic—and encouraging. Remember to
praise yourself for gradual changes. If exercise has been an aversive
topic to you in the past, you may need to review this chapter several
times and to read some of the evidence first-hand. Sometimes old
myths are comfortable—and stubborn. It may be extremely important
initially for you to tune in to your monologues about exercise—and to
revise them if they need it. You may need to cue yourself to avoid step
saving. You must train yourself to *think* many times a day: how can I
accomplish this task and comfortably spend more calories in the process?

   Your physical environment may also need some rearranging.
Your house or office may now be arranged for "convenience." That
translates into "work saving." Arranging your physical surroundings
a little more inconveniently may help you spend many more calories.
Consider the possibility of having one or more of your extension
phones removed. Buy small wastebaskets that demand more frequent
emptying. Scout out your environment for physical devices or arrange-

ments that contribute to step saving. Obviously, you do not want to eliminate all the objects that make life easier. Look for revisions in your physical setup that would be easy to live with while increasing calorie spending.

Finally, your social environment may need attention. Involve your family as extensively as possible in your efforts to become an activist. Seek their support—and by all means, compliment it! Your efforts may benefit them in the long run. If you plan to establish a special exercise routine in addition to expanding your daily activity, try to plan it with a friend. Shared activity is often more enjoyable; it also means you have a commitment to keep your exercise appointments. Consider the possibility of increasing the activity level of some of your social interactions. A formal dinner party is hardly the place to begin. Picnics, cookouts, and other informal social occasions are a different matter. Picnics often consist of eating and sitting! Take a walk; throw a frisbee; play a game. Be the initiator of *fun* activities for your social group.

You have been exposed to a great deal of information in this chapter. Do not hesitate to review as extensively as is necessary for a clear understanding of this important topic. Remember as you tackle your exercise habits: you don't have to exhaust yourself to expend calories. Regular, moderate exercise involving gross body movements is most effective in weight control.

ASSIGNMENT 5

If you have a good grasp of the principles involved in energy expenditure and the guidelines for increasing your calorie spending, you are ready to evaluate and improve your status as an activist. We recommend that you spend a minimum of four weeks on this assignment—and longer if you are not *very* confident that your exercise habits are improving satisfactorily. Your evaluation of your progress should be based on *behavior change*. Remember: your progress will be faster and more permanent if you concentrate on behavior changed (e.g., activity increased) rather than weight lost. Don't expect overnight success. You can be confident that concentration on moderate restriction of caloric intake combined with moderate exercise *will* eliminate unwanted pounds. Change your patterns, and you will lose weight.

Stage 1: Specify area. The area of concern, of course, is your activity level. Remember that your exercise habits can affect *both* sides of the energy equation. The activist gets double returns—provided that the principles we've discussed are utilized in increasing and maintaining activity level. In this assignment, you will be evaluating *your* exercise habits, assessing *your* activity level.

Stage 2: Collect data. The recommended data collection strategy for this assignment differs from the others you will be given. Even a moment's consideration suggests that collecting data on your activity level is rather difficult—especially since we *urge* you to focus primarily on your daily routine. Recording "time spent actively" is virtually impossible; you would be spending most of your working hours with a stopwatch in hand! Recording the number of times you perform certain tasks is also an ineffective data collection system. Think of the list of activities this would entail. Both these systems are much too cumbersome and time-consuming.

Yet the importance of accurate activity data cannot be overemphasized. As we have noted, most sedentary individuals do not perceive themselves as sedentary. It is very easy to equate fatigue or a busy schedule with calorie expenditure. *Accurate data in this area are very important.* There is a simple, efficient, and accurate data collection device available, and we strongly recommend that you purchase one. This device is called a *pedometer;* it measures distance covered in miles. As you know from the section on principles of expenditure, this is an excellent measure of energy expended. A pedometer provides a convenient system for obtaining quantifiable data. It is a small device about the size of a stopwatch that can be easily (and inconspicuously) attached to a pocket or belt. It can be purchased at most sporting goods stores at a cost of $10 to $13. If you are reluctant to spend money on a device that you are unfamiliar with, your attitude is understandable. You should consider, however, the long-term advantages of effective weight control and weigh them against $10. We can assure you it is money well spent.

We recommend the following system for collecting and recording your data. *As soon as you get up* each morning, set your pedometer at 0 and attach it to yourself at the hip or ankle. At noon each day, record the reading from the pedometer, which will be the distance you have traveled during the morning. Then reset your pedometer at 0. At dinner time, again check your pedometer and record the reading, which is the distance you have covered in the afternoon. Again, reset the pedometer to 0. At bedtime, follow the same procedure. Record the reading from your pedometer (distance covered in the evening). Now, add the three readings for the day—the total distance you covered during that day. Try to record your data at the same time each day, for example, at 12:00, 6:00 p.m., and 11:00 p.m.

We recommend that you make up and use a form like the following:

ACTIVITY RECORD

Total Miles

Week _____   Covered _____

	Mon.	Tues.	Wed.	Thurs.	Fri.	Sat.	Sun.
Morning	½ mi.						
Afternoon	¾ mi.						
Evening	¼ mi.						
Total	1½ mi.						

FIGURE 6

Let's take a particular day as an example. On Monday morning, as soon as you are out of bed, you set your pedometer at 0 and put it on. At noon you check it; it reads ½ mile. Record that in the Monday morning block. Reset the pedometer to 0.

At 6:00 p.m., you check again. This time the reading is ¾ mile. Record that in the Monday afternoon block. Reset to 0. At 11:00 p.m. (or bedtime), again check and record your data. This time the pedometer reads ¼ mile. Record that in the Monday evening block. Now, total your amounts for the day and record in the "total" block. For this particular day, your total distance covered was 1½ miles.

This system is both convenient and simple; it provides excellent data on your activity level. Try to record at the same time each day, and be sure to remember to reset your pedometer to 0 each time you record. You should collect data for one full week before continuing.

STOP! DO NOT READ ON UNTIL
YOU HAVE COMPLETED STAGE 2

3. *Identify patterns.* At the end of one week—if it is a fairly typical week—you should have a reasonably accurate picture of your status as an activist. If your week has been atypical, by all means continue recording for another full week.

Let's see what your data suggest. If you are walking less than two miles per day (*especially* if you are female), inactivity is *very* likely to be a major component in your weight problem. If you are covering two to four miles per day, it probably needs some improvement. If you are covering five or more miles per day, it is *less* likely to be a problem component—but do not rule it out too quickly. Research suggests that most nonobese males and females walk approximately four to five miles per day.

Let's assume your daily average is under five miles. What patterns can you detect by inspecting your data? Are your mornings consistently much more sedentary than your afternoons? Is your activity level in the evenings lower than either? Is a certain day's activity level much higher than other days? What about weekends—how do they compare with weekdays?

Now, compare your data to your daily routine. Is a certain day your laundry day—involving several trips up and down the basement steps? Is your total higher on housecleaning day? This type of comparison can tell you fairly specifically just where your sedentary spots are. Maybe you need to increase your morning activity. Possibly weekends need to become a little more active. Glean as much information as you can from your data; it's an invaluable aid in effective problem solving.

Now, what if your data indicate you are covering five or more miles per day? Don't make hasty judgments. It is still possible that your activity level needs increasing. However, it is certainly advisable to check the other half of the energy equation—your caloric intake. Remember—the best strategy is a combination of moderation on both sides. If your activity level is moderate to high (five miles and up per day), you should emphasize modifying your intake more extensively.

Experiment, keeping in mind the principles you've learned and your personal data.

4. *Examine options.* If you are in the two to four mile per day range, you need to become more active. There are two general options for increasing your activity level—you can make your daily routine more active; in addition, you can establish a regular pattern of more vigorous "extracurricular" exercise, such as swimming, etc. Note that we said, "in addition." We strongly encourage you to pursue the former option of adjusting your daily activities even if you also decide to work on the latter.

A very good option to pursue initially is that of revising your environments. What can you do to improve your exercise ecology? How are your activity attitudes? It might be helpful initially (until your new calorie spending attitude becomes habit) to post some reminders in conspicuous places, reminders that your new goal is to take *more* steps. Your goal is to plan your day with the question constantly in mind: how can I spend more calories in doing this differently? These reminders will cue different behaviors; they will also ease you into thinking differently about exercise. Regardless of what specific options you choose, watch your goals. Increase your "distance covered" gradually. Make sure your increases fall within your comfort zone. If feelings and thoughts about the aversiveness of your strategies crop up, change your strategies!

Involve your family in your efforts as extensively as possible. Their support will be invaluable. However, if they are not supportive, it is not catastrophic. Their cooperation and praise would be helpful, but your activity level is up to you. Even if they don't appreciate your efforts, you should. Plan to tell yourself frequently that you do.

Program your physical surroundings to increase your activity. A good idea may be to walk through your house with a notebook, jotting down ideas as you go. In each room you should ask: what arrangements and devices in this room save me steps? Now, which ones could I rearrange or eliminate without making life aversive? Remember: you're looking for changes that will increase calorie spending fairly comfortably. Life doesn't have to be backbreaking to be active. Make as long a list as you can. Then choose several options from it. Keep your list for later adjustments. Could you do without that extension phone? What about moving your garbage cans a little farther from the door? What about rearranging your office a little more inconveniently? Can you increase your trips up and down your stairway by moving some items up or down? Remember to consider your family as you plan changes in your physical environment. Unless they are very cooperative or have joined you in your reduction efforts, they may object to changes which make more work for them.

Utilize your data in examining other options. Look at your patterns. If mornings are consistently active but afternoons consistently sedentary, think about your typical afternoon routine. Does it emphasize reading, watching television, sitting at your desk? What can you do to activate it? Could commercials serve as a cue for activity? Water your plants; walk upstairs a time or two; empty the garbage—even if it's only half full; walk the dog. Set a timer for every 20 or 30 minutes; take a quick walk through your house (or around it) each time it rings. Break up those long sedentary stretches.

There are countless ways to accomplish the general goal of calorie spending. Stand, walk, bend, move! Even shifting your weight from one leg to the other is better than nothing. Think of as many options as you can so that you can have some variety in choice.

5. *Narrow and experiment.* Select four or five specific options from your list. You might try to choose some that involve physical rearrangement; definitely choose some that involve different ways of performing the same tasks you usually perform (stair climbing versus elevator riding, etc.).

As you plan your strategies, remember the principles you have learned. Increase activities that involve large muscle masses. Move your body through distances. Work against gravity; climb stairs!

If you choose to increase extra activities, make sure they're pleasurable. Ask a friend to join you.

Continue the same recording system you have begun. In addition, keep a list (possibly posted as a reminder) of the changes you are working on.

6. *Compare data.* As always, when you compare data, concentrate on behaviors changed, not pounds lost. Check your daily averages; also look for success spots and weak spots. Do mornings look better? Compare your new data with your previous data as specifically as possible. Look for the places in which changes have and have not occurred.

7. *Extend, revise, or replace.* We recommend that you spend a minimum of three weeks total in actual implementation of your strategies. Compare your data (and revise your strategies if necessary) approximately every four or five days. It may be difficult to estimate ahead of time how much change certain strategies will produce. There is no reason to spend a week on the same options if for four days running they only raised your daily total by 1/16 of a mile! On the other hand, you need to allow approximately four days for fairly accurate evalution. Daily variations will occur.

Have the options you've chosen increased your daily miles by an average of ½ mile or more per day? Initially that is adequate. You may be aiming for several more miles per day, but not all at once. Are you comfortable with your strategies? Are some *too* strenuous? Now, what else can you add to increase your activity for the next four or five days?

Remember to change your options to prevent boredom; continue looking for new ways to be more active. Don't be afraid to experiment.

We suggest you wear a pedometer and collect data for at least six weeks. You should wear it for at least two weeks after you have reached a comfortably more active daily routine. Check yourself frequently after you've reached your goal; wear your pedometer for one full day every two weeks for a period of several months.

Becoming an activist can be fun—if you remember that you are working on establishing lifetime habits. Expecting perfection leads to frustration. *Anticipate* that you will need to revise and change your strategies for greater effectiveness and for variety.

11
Emotional Eating:
Relax—You're Not Hungry

Many people report that they eat whenever they become anxious, depressed, lonely, or tired. There are several possible reasons for this problematical pattern.

To begin with, most of us are very poor labelers. The internal physiological feelings of anxiety and depression are often very hard to distinguish from those of hunger. For example, two people may both feel tired, lightheaded, weak, and somewhat tense. One of them may attribute these sensations to air pollution, a seasonal virus, poor sleeping habits, or the sight of the kids' school bus. The second may inadvertently label these sensations as "hunger." Physiological research over the last decade has suggested that many individuals—and particularly those who are overweight—have difficulty distinguishing hunger from other states of physiological arousal. Unfortunately, this may mean that the overweight individual eats in response to a variety of mistaken internal cues. In a sense, he may have become a poor labeler of his own private environment.

A second possible reason for the frequency of eating in response to tension, anxiety, and depression is that eating has long been associated with anxiety reduction. Food does help to alleviate tension. Most parents capitalize on this principle when they use milk or sweets to soothe a child. Unfortunately, the pattern can easily become a problematical one. As the child grows up, he learns to associate food with anxiety reduction—fattening sweets become a dangerous "pick-me-up" or relaxant.

Some individuals report that they overeat in order to punish themselves for their misdeeds. Ironically, those misdeeds are often acts of overeating! A perfectionistic dieter may "sin" by eating a forbidden fruit. The guilt, anxiety, and depression which follow are sometimes cues for further eating—which, in turn, leads to further depression.

These vicious cycles are not an infrequent component in obesity. Unless they are interrupted and corrected, they can lead to a long and miserable sequence.

ILLUSTRATION

Mr. Reynolds was a 45-year-old businessman who had been overweight since childhood. He worked an average of 50 hours per week and his days were generally very hectic.

Stage 1: Specify area. Upon learning about the possible role of emotional eating in obesity, Mr. Reynolds decided to examine whether his own eating habits were influenced by anxiety.

Stage 2: Collect data. He bought a small notebook and divided each page into three parts:

Anxious Before?	Eating Incident	Anxious After?

FIGURE 7

Whenever he ate, Mr. Reynolds wrote a brief description under the column marked "Eating Incident." If he had been anxious or tense prior to eating, he wrote "Yes" in the left column. Similarly, in the right column he indicated whether he was still anxious after he had eaten. A sample day's record is shown below.

Anxious Before?	Eating Incident		Anxious After?
No	8:00	Breakfast	No
Yes	10:00	Snack (doughnut)	Yes
Yes	12:30	Lunch	No
Yes	2:30	Snack (candy)	Yes
Yes	5:15	Drink (martini)	No
No	6:30	Dinner	No

FIGURE 8

Notice that Mr. Reynolds' record system might have overlooked some important factors in his eating patterns. For example, he monitored only anxious eating and might accidentally have overlooked boredom eating or the "pick-me-up" eating sometimes used to cope with depression.

Stage 3: Identify patterns. Despite the possible flaws in his record keeping system, after one week Mr. Reynolds had discovered some very important regularities in his behavior. First, he was, in fact, often tense or anxious before he ate. This was particularly true when he snacked or drank. Thus, emotional eating was indeed a possible element in his weight problem. A second discovery was that most of his nervous eating occurred at work rather than at home. Finally, he noticed that—for him—eating didn't seem to be a very effective antidote for tension. Half of the time he was just as anxious *after* eating as he had been before.

Stage 4: Examine options. Mr. Reynolds listed the following as possible solutions:

a. begin taking tranquilizers at work;
b. take lower calorie snacks to work;
c. change jobs;
d. learn to be less tense at work;
e. learn to do something other than eat when you are tense.

Stage 5: Narrow and experiment. He decided that changing jobs was unfeasible and that tranquilizers were not a pleasant alternative. Taking lower calorie snacks to work had some potential, but his secretary often brought sweets and there was a candy machine in the lobby of his office building. Mr. Reynolds therefore decided to try learning to be more relaxed in his work environment. He experimented with a set of relaxation exercises (which are provided in your next assignment). He practiced the exercises at home each day for one week. During the second week, he placed a kitchen timer in his desk at the office and set it for one hour intervals. Each time it rang, he evaluated his tension and practiced a brief version of the exercises.

Stage 6: Compare data. Mr. Reynolds found the relaxation assignment very helpful in dealing with his anxious eating. Practicing at work—in the midst of his hectic daily pressures—was particularly successful. His records showed a dramatic decline in the frequency of emotional eating.

Stage 7: Extend, revise, or replace. Mr. Reynolds decided to continue his relaxation strategy and to broaden its application. He bought a portable parking meter timer to carry in his pocket when he left the office. Whenever it buzzed, he monitored his tension level and, if necessary, took a few moments to relax himself. After four weeks, he discontinued his recording of anxious eating with the understanding that he would resume it every once in a while to evaluate his progress and resolve any problem developments.

Relaxation training is not the only strategy which has been used successfully in helping people to resolve anxiety or boredom eating. However, it has been one of the most consistently effective. Whether it works for you, of course, can only be determined by a personal experiment. In your next assignment you will be given detailed guidelines for relaxation exercises along with some alternative options for reducing eating in response to stress. First, however, you need to determine whether emotional eating is a problem for you.

ASSIGNMENT 6

Stage 1: Specify area. Are you an emotional eater? Do you often use foods as a "pick-me-up" or as something to do when you are bored? Can you recall recent instances in which you ate in response to tension?

Stage 2: Collect data. For the next week, monitor the emotions which precede your eating. Devise a record keeping system like Mr. Reynold's and prepare a week's worth of forms. To avoid overlooking depression or boredom eating, change the column headings in your forms to "Emotion Before," "Eating Incident," and "Emotion After." Try to describe your feelings accurately in a single word like "angry," "lonely," and so on. Be sure to carry your diary with you so you can record instances as they occur. Remember, immediate recording is important—your memory often plays tricks on you when you try to recall patterns hours after they have occurred.

STOP! DO NOT READ ON UNTIL YOU HAVE COMPLETED STAGE 2.

Stage 3: Identify patterns. What do your records suggest? How often did you eat in response to tension or negative emotions? Were many different emotions associated with eating? How effective was eating in coping with your feelings? Were there any patterns in the timing of your nervous eating (evenings, weekends, etc.)? How about location?

If your records showed very little emotional eating, consider their accuracy before you skip to the next chapter. Did you monitor for at least one week? Are you confident of the accuracy of your record keeping? Were there other factors which may have reduced problem eating during the week? If so, you may want to complete some further observations or practice the exercises outlined below. However, if you are fairly confident that emotional eating is not a problem for you, go on to the next chapter.

Stage 4: Examine options. Let's temporarily ignore the fact that you will soon be given instructions on how to relax yourself. What are the other options? Can you make changes in your physical environment? Your social environment? Your private environment? Developing alternative responses to tension, anger, and boredom, of course, is the major purpose of relaxation exercises. However, in this assignment and all others, it is critically important that you have several options available. Even though relaxation training has helped a large number of people, you have to be prepared for the possibility that it may not help you. Remember, the most meaningful data in your reduction efforts are your own. Specify what you will do if the exercises below are not effective in reducing your emotional eating. Meditation and deep-breathing exercises are two alternatives you might consider.

Stage 5: Narrow and experiment. Since relaxation exercises have been a popular and frequently successful strategy in dealing with emotional eating, let's assume that they are your first choice. Remember to continue monitoring your emotional eating for the next two weeks so that you can evaluate the effects of your self-experiment.

RELAXATION EXERCISES

For greatest effectiveness, the exercises described below should be read to you very slowly by a friend or spouse. An alternative would be to tape record them so that they can be played back whenever you desire. You can, of course, record them yourself. This removes the need for you to read the exercises each time you practice. Reading may distract your attention and reduce the degree of relaxation attained.

In going through the exercises, use voice quality and volume to contrast relaxation with tension. That is, when you are instructed to tense a muscle, the instruction should be given in a relatively loud, high-pitched voice. Instructions to relax should first be given loudly and later in a softer, lower-pitched voice. To assist you or your helper in this distinction, *italics indicate where a soft, soothing voice should be used.*

The full list of exercises takes about 30 to 40 minutes. If you finish before then, your pacing is probably too fast. Practice the exercises once per day for five days. Then try to abbreviate them so that you can relax in a shorter period of time without having to tense all of the muscles in the original exercises. With two weeks of daily practice you should be able to relax yourself in a few minutes without having to tense any muscles at all. During the second week of your experiment, *practice your relaxation skills in the actual situations which often lead to emotional eating.*

Before you begin these exercises, find a comfortable chair or place to lie down. It should be relatively quiet and only dimly lighted. Remove any tight pieces of clothing such as your shoes. If you wear glasses or contact lenses, they should be removed. Dentures should also be removed and you should try to assume a position which is as comfortable as possible for you. A lounge chair, lying on the couch, and lying on a bed are ideal. If you like, however, an easy chair is sufficient.

When you do assume a comfortable position, make sure that you are supporting as little of your body as possible. That is, let the bed or chair or couch hold as much of your weight as it possibly can. You don't want to have to hold your head up with your neck muscles, and you don't want to be slouching in a chair so that the muscles in your lower back will become sore.

Once you have assumed a comfortable position we can begin exercising some of the muscle groups and training you to become familiar with the signs of anxiety and muscular tension. In addition, you will learn how to turn on a relaxed sensation in your muscles. We will do this by first tensing and then relaxing some of the major muscles in your body. You will be asked to tense them and to concentrate on the tension for two to three seconds. You will then be told to relax them. When the word "Relax" is presented, you should immediately let the muscles become as limp as possible and focus on the sensations which you then feel. This will allow you to become more familiar with what it feels like to be muscularly tense and anxious. You will also gain skills in being able to detect these cues and to change the muscular tension into a form of relaxation.

To begin, clench your right fist as tight as you possibly can. Clench the fist until you feel the tension in your fingers and along the knuckles. Hold that tension. You should be tensing it so tight that your hand is almost shaking. Concentrate on that tension, hold it there, and now RELAX and *let your fingers drop very limply. They will passively stretch out and lengthen. You will feel the muscles loosen up. Focus on the sensation of relaxation which you now feel in your right hand. There is a warm, soothing sensation as the muscles relax, and you should contrast that relaxing sensation to the tension.* Remaining as relaxed as possible in other parts of your body, again tense your right fist. Clench the fist as tightly as possible. Concentrate on the tension. Hold it there . . . hold it . . . and RELAX. *Let the hand go limp. Now concentrate on that relaxed sensation. It is that warm, soothing, relaxed feeling that you would like to overtake your entire body.*

This time we are going to clench both fists at the same time. Clench both your right and left hands as tightly as you can. Concentrate on the tension. Tighter . . . tighter . . . and RELAX. *Let both hands go limp; let the fingers stretch out very passively. You will feel a warm, soothing sensation. Now focus on what it feels like to have your hands as relaxed as possible.*

At different times throughout these exercises you will be asked to take a deep breath. When requested, inhale as deeply as possible, hold your breath for about one second, and then exhale very, very slowly at your own pace. As you exhale slowly you should try to relax as much as possible. Try to relax even deeper and let the air out as gradually as you can. All right . . . take a deep breath—as deep as you can. Hold it for one second . . . *and now exhale very, very slowly. As you exhale you want to RELAX as much as you can. Very relaxed . . . let the muscles go.*

We are now going to move up the arm into some of the other major muscles. As we move on to these other muscle groups, you should try to keep your hands and wrists as relaxed as you possibly can. The next muscles that we are going to work on are in the forearm. Your arms should be lying very comfortably at your sides. If you are sitting in a chair they may be resting either on your lap or on the arms of the chair. We are going to begin by exercising some of the muscles in the front of your forearm. To do this, keep your fingers relaxed but bend both of your hands at the wrist so that your palms are facing away from you. Pull your fingers toward your face and concentrate on the sensations in your forearms. Focus on that tension . . . hold them . . . and RELAX. *Let your hands resume a comfortable position. Now focus on that warm, relaxed feeling in your wrists and forearms. Very relaxed . . . very soothing.*

We are now going to work on the opposing muscle group in the forearm. Again, keep your fingers as relaxed as possible. This time bend both hands at the wrist so that the palms are facing toward you. Pull your fingers in toward your body. Concentrate on the tension in the outer part of your forearm. Pull those fingers in. Hold it there . . . and RELAX. *Let the hands resume a normal, comfortable position. Allow the muscles to lengthen very slowly. RELAX. Very passive. Focus your attention on that warm, soothing feeling in the forearm muscles.*

We can now move on to the muscles in the upper arm. We will first work on the biceps, the large muscle in the front of your upper arm. Let's begin by exercising your right arm only. Leave your left arm as relaxed as possible and try to maintain relaxed feelings in the fingers and forearms of both arms. Bend your right arm at the elbow so that you are bringing your hand up toward your shoulder. Make a muscle with your biceps. To do that you may actually have to touch your shoulder with your hand, but you should feel tension in the upper part of your arm, the front of your arm. Concentrate on that tension . . . tense the biceps . . . and RELAX. *Let your arm resume a normal, comfortable position. It should fall very limply and lightly. The relaxed feeling in your right biceps should be very noticeable.* Remember to keep your forearms and fingers as relaxed as possible as you go through these upper arm exercises.

This time let's do it with your left arm. Bend your left arm at the elbow so that your left hand is almost touching your shoulder. Concentrate on flexing the left biceps. Concentrate on the tension . . . hold it there . . . and RELAX. *Let your arm resume a comfortable position. Very relaxed. Focus your attention on that warm, soothing sensation in the muscle. You would like that sensation to spread throughout your arms and eventually throughout the rest of your body.*

Let's go back to the right arm again. This time we will be exercising the triceps muscle, which is the back part of your upper arm. In order to flex this muscle you have to straighten your arm out. You should try to keep your wrist and forearm as relaxed as possible but you will be straightening your arm out so that there is no angle at the elbow. If you like you can actually push back against something. In a chair, for example, you can let your arm dangle over the side and push backwards against one of the rear chair legs. On a bed you can just push straight down and feel tension in the muscle in the back part of your upper arm. Find a position where you can produce tension in your right triceps. Flex that muscle . . . concentrate on the tension . . . push as hard as you can . . . push it . . . and RELAX. *Let your arm relax as much as you can. Focus on that warm, relaxed sensation in the upper arm muscles and let that relaxed sensation spread throughout the arm.*

Now let's move over to the left arm. Again find something that you can push against so that you can produce tension in that left triceps muscle. Flex the muscle . . . concentrate on the tension . . . push . . . and RELAX. *Let the arm resume a comfortable position. Relax as much as possible. Focus your attention on that warm, relaxed feeling.*

Take a very deep breath. Hold it for one second and as you exhale very slowly, relax as much as you can. Take a deep breath . . . as you exhale RELAX . . . RELAX. *Let all the muscles become as relaxed as you can. You want to smooth them out.*

We are next going to relax some of the other muscle groups. As we do, you should try to keep your forearms, hands, and upper arm muscles as relaxed as possible. Try not to tense them any more. First of all, let's exercise some of the muscles in the shoulders and upper back. Shrug your shoulders in a very exaggerated fashion. Bring both of your shoulders up towards your ears . . . hold them as high as you can . . . higher . . . hold them . . . and RELAX. *Let your shoulders resume a comfortable position. Now concentrate on that warm, relaxed feeling in the shoulder muscles and along the upper part of your back. A very soothing sensation. You should make a mental note of what it feels like to have those muscles relaxed so that in the future you can turn on this relaxed feeling without having to tense them.* Concentrate on that warm, relaxed feeling.

Next we are going to work on some of the muscles in the neck. Start turning your head very slowly to the right. Turn it very slowly until you reach a point where you can't turn it anymore. When you get to that point, gently push a little bit further. You will feel tension along the left side of your neck. Push a little more . . . feel that tension . . . push . . . and RELAX. *Let the neck muscles smooth out. Allow your head to resume a comfortable position and concentrate on that very warm and pleasant sensation in the neck muscles.*

We will now exercise the opposing muscle groups. This time turn your head very slowly to the left. Very slowly, until you reach that sticking point. When you reach that point, push a little bit further until you feel tension along the right side of your neck. Push until you feel that tension . . . hold it there . . . hold it . . . and RELAX. *Let the muscles smooth out and concentrate on that warm, relaxed feeling.*

Next, we are going up into some of the facial muscles. These are extremely important in terms of everyday tension and anxiety. You should take your time here and nake sure that you can focus on what it feels like to relax these muscles. To begin with we will work with the jaw muscles and the muscles around the mouth. Open your mouth as wide as you possibly can. Open it as wide as you can. Hold it open as far as you can . . . concentrate on the tension in the jaw muscles . . . and RELAX. *Let your mouth resume a comfortable position and focus on the sensations along your jaw muscles. As they smooth out, they assume a passive, relaxed state and you feel a warm, pleasant sensation.*

To exercise the opposing muscle group, close your mouth and bite down on the molars in the back of the mouth so that you are biting down as hard as you can. Concentrate on the tension in your jaws. Bite down as hard as you can . . . hold it there . . . and RELAX. *Let the muscles relax as much as they can. They should smooth out and you should feel no tension whatsoever in the muscles along your jaw and around your mouth.*

We are now going to exercise a slightly different set of muscles around the mouth. This time don't bring your teeth together but close your lips and exaggerate a grin. Keep your lips closed but bring the corners of your mouth up as high as you can toward your eyes. Bring the corners of your mouth up as high as you can. Concentrate on the tension in your cheeks and in the muscles around your mouth. Hold it there . . . and RELAX.

Let the muscles resume a comfortable position. Take a few moments to focus on that warm, relaxed feeling in these muscles.

Take a very deep breath . . . hold it for one second . . . and exhale very slowly. As you exhale, allow yourself to go deeper and deeper into a relaxed state.

We are next going to exercise some of the muscles around the eyes. These are again very important in handling the tension of everyday situations. Be sure to focus your attention on what it feels like to tense and relax these muscles. To begin, open both eyes as wide as you possibly can. Bring the eyebrows up as high as possible and pull the cheek muscles down. You should be opening your eyes as much as you can . . . hold it there . . . concentrate on that tension . . . and RELAX. *Let the muscles smooth out. Let your eyes resume a comfortable position and simply focus on the sensations that you now feel around the eye muscles.*

Using the opposing muscle group, close your eyes as tightly as you possibly can. Bring the eyeballs down and your cheek muscles up as tight as you can. You may even see stars. Tighten them as much as you can . . . concentrate on that tension . . . hold it there . . . and RELAX. *Let the muscles relax and focus on that warm, pleasant sensation you feel when you relax the muscles around the eyes.* You may find it comfortable simply to let your eyelids close. This allows you to pay more attention to these pleasant sensations.

One final muscle group that we will be working on in the facial area involves the muscles in your forehead. These muscles are again very important in what most people consider tension or muscular anxiety. You will frequently find after you practice these exercises that the forehead muscles are often those which tense first in anxiety situations. Pay particular attention to what it feels like to relax these muscles so that you will then be cued in everyday situations when you start becoming tense. In order to flex these muscles, wrinkle your forehead as much as you can and pull your nose muscles up toward your eyes. You should be pulling the forehead muscles down to form an exaggerated scowl. There are quite a few muscle groups involved here. Concentrate on tensing as many of them as you can . . . hold it there . . . hold it . . . and RELAX. *Concentrate on the warm, relaxed sensation.*

Take a few moments right now to inventory the muscles around your face. If any of them feel tense, try to relax away the tension without again flexing the muscles. Concentrate on the muscles of the forehead, around the eyes, and the jaw muscles. If you feel any tension whatsoever, try to relax it away so that all the muscles feel very smooth . . . very placid . . . and very relaxed.

Let's take a moment here to inventory the progress we have made. *Focus on the sensations in your shoulders. If you feel any tension there, relax it away. Now slowly guide your concentration down into the arms. They should be very comfortable. The upper arms should be very relaxed, both the front and back. Your forearms and the fingers should feel very limp and heavy. All of the muscles should be smoothed out and relaxed.* If you feel any tension whatsoever in these muscles, take a few seconds now to relax it slowly away. Continue the exercises below only when you have reached a calm, passive relaxation in your arms, shoulders, neck, and facial muscles.

Take a deep breath, hold it for one second, and *as you exhale very slowly, concentrate on becoming more and more relaxed. Let all the muscles smooth out and eliminate every bit of tension from your body.*

The next muscle group we will work with involves the abdominal muscles and some of the muscles in the chest and trunk region. As you exercise these areas, try to keep the rest of your body as relaxed as possible. Remember, your shoulders, neck, arms, and facial muscles should remain as relaxed as possible from here on out. Now then, tense the muscles in the stomach area by pushing them out. You are trying to make a ball with your stomach. Push the muscles out and round your stomach as much as you can. Concentrate on the tension as you push the muscles out . . . hold it there . . . and RELAX. *Let the muscles relax and concentrate on that warm sensation as they smooth out. You want to focus on what it feels like to relax those muscles and again allow that warm, pleasant sensation to spread to other areas in your body so that all of your muscles are as relaxed as possible.*

This time pull your stomach muscles in as much as possible. Pull them in so you are trying to touch your abdomen to your backbone. Pull them in as much as possible . . . feel that tension in the muscles . . . hold it there . . . and RELAX. *Let the muscles smooth out. Let that soothing, relaxed feeling overtake all of the muscles in the abdominal area, and allow yourself to sink deeper and deeper into this warm pool of relaxation. The muscles should feel very heavy, very limp—as if they were just hanging there.* You are doing nothing to support them. They are as relaxed as they can possibly be.

We are now going to move on to the muscles in your legs. As we work on these exercises, remember to keep your upper body, your arms, and your facial muscles as relaxed as you possibly can. We shall begin with the muscles in the upper part of your right leg. In order to exercise those muscles, stretch out your right leg so that you have straightened it and you have locked your knee. When you lock the knee push a little further and you will feel tension in the upper part of your right leg, particularly in the top part of the muscle. Stretch it so that you feel that tension. Tense it as much as possible. Hold it there . . . concentrate on the tension in the leg . . . and RELAX. *Let your leg resume a comfortable position and focus your attention on what it feels like to relax those large muscles in the upper leg.*

This time let's work on the muscle in the upper part of your left leg. Again straighten the leg out until you have locked the knee. Once you have locked the knee, tense the muscle in the upper part of the leg as much as you can. Concentrate on tensing that muscle . . . hold it there . . . hold it . . . and RELAX. *Let the muscles smooth out and concentrate on that warm, pleasant sensation. Allow that sensation to spread throughout the upper leg area so that you feel no tension whatsoever.*

Moving back to the right leg, we are now going to exercise the muscles in the calf area. Remember we are working only on the right leg now. Begin to push your toes away from you as if you were pushing down on a gas pedal. Push the toes away from you as far as you can. The muscles in your toes, in the ball of your foot, and in the calf area should feel very tense. Concentrate on pushing as much as you can. Tense those muscles . . . hold it there . . . and RELAX. *Let the muscles smooth out. Concentrate on what it feels like to relax those muscles.*

Now let's do it with the left leg. With the left leg only, push the toes away from you as far as you can until you feel tension in the ball of your left foot and in your left calf. Push as hard as you can . . . push even further . . . push . . . and RELAX. *Let the muscles smooth out and concentrate on allowing yourself to relax deeper and deeper so you feel no tension whatsoever in your legs. They feel very heavy and limp.*

Now let's try it with both feet at the same time. Push with both feet. Push the toes away from you and pull the heels up toward you. Feel that tension in the calf muscles and the balls of your feet. Hold it there . . . concentrate on the tension . . . and RELAX. *Let them smooth out. Let the muscles relax as much as possible and focus your attention on those sensations.*

We are now going to exercise an opposing muscle group. Again let's use both legs at one time. However, instead of pushing the toes away from you, this time you should pull them toward you. Pull your toes upward and the heels should be going away from you. It is as if you are trying to lift a weight with your toes alone. You should be pulling your toes toward your knees. Concentrate on producing as much tension as you can in the calf area and in the lower part of your ankles. Feel tension in both feet. Pull the toes toward you . . . concentrate on that tension . . . hold it there . . . and RELAX. *Let the feet resume a comfortable position and concentrate on those warm, pleasant sensations as all of the muscles in the calf, ankle, and foot areas relax, smooth out, and assume a very warm, heavy, limp state.*

Take a deep breath, hold it for one second, and *as you exhale very slowly, concentrate on becoming more and more relaxed.* Try to let yourself smooth all of the muscles out. You should feel no tension whatsoever.

Take a very slow inventory starting with your feet and moving up your body from one section to the next. If you feel any tension whatsoever, try to relax it away without tensing the muscles. *Just allow that warm, pleasant, relaxed feeling to spread from one section to the next so that all of the muscles are very smooth . . . very relaxed. You should now have no tension in the feet . . . in the calves . . . in the upper legs . . . the abdomen area . . . chest . . . shoulders . . . neck . . . jaws . . . muscles around the eyes . . . the forehead . . . your upper arms . . . forearms . . . and hands. All of the muscles are very relaxed . . . they have smoothed out . . . and you feel no tension. Take a few seconds here to allow yourself to sink even deeper. If you are lying on a bed or sitting on a chair, allow yourself to sink even deeper. All of your weight should be supported by the couch, or bed, or chair. Your entire body should be limp and very relaxed.*

These exercises provide you with excellent training in what it feels like to be relaxed and what the cues are for muscular tension. As you practice the exercises you should try to anticipate yourself somewhat so that you can learn to relax the muscles without even tensing them. Eventually you will be able to produce a very relaxed feeling in the major muscle groups within a matter of seconds. And even more important, you will start to pick up cues of muscular tension in everyday situations. These cues can be signals to you that you should take a few moments and relax yourself. You should also get into the habit of taking brief muscle inventories to find out whether you are muscularly tense in certain situations. Get in the habit of relaxing those muscles you do not need for a particular task. For example, you may notice that as you drive you often tense many muscles which are unnecessary for good driving skills. In that situation, try to relax all of those muscles which do not need to be tense—such as the facial or forehead muscles. Try to relax yourself as much as possible without turning off the muscles you need for the task at hand.

As you become more skilled in this relaxation technique, you will find that it can be applied in many different situations in your daily life. Several of our clients have found relaxation skills very helpful in enabling them to cope with a variety of problems and fears in addition to emotional eating. Insomnia, fear of public speaking, fear of flying—all these have been alleviated by relaxation training.

Stage 6: Compare data. Do your self-records indicate any change in emotional eating? Are there some situations which have improved and others which have not? Did you practice the exercises conscientiously? How successful were they in making you feel relaxed? If your efforts were diligent but minimally successful, consider some alternatives such as those suggested earlier (page 151).

Stage 7: Extend, revise, or replace. If your experiment showed some promise or you feel the need for further relaxation practice, continue your exercises as before. Remember to work toward an abbreviated strategy in which you can relax yourself in a matter of minutes without tensing muscles.

If your experiment was not promising and you feel confident in your data and adherence to the assignment, consider possible options. Were there any factors which prevented your learning to relax? Could you practice relaxation in different situations? Which of the other options might be helpful in place of relaxation?

12
Troubleshooting and Maintenance

If you have followed our recommended sequence of apprenticeship in personal science, you are now—several months later—a veteran problem solver. While your self-control skills may still leave room for improvement, they are probably much more versatile and efficient. In a very real sense, the worst part of your reducing battle should be over. You should have taken considerable pride in both your commitment and your progress. The emerging "new you" is not only thinner and healthier—it is also more confident and capable.

As we mentioned at the beginning of the book, successful weight control must be measured in terms of permanence. Your hard-fought battle would be all but meaningless if you could have no assurance of lifelong benefits. You should now be well aware of the health dangers inherent in temporary diets and relapses.

The skills you have learned as a personal scientist will provide you with the best possible chances of continued progress and enduring maintenance. This does not mean that you can complacently declare the war over and slip into an "off my diet" stance. Self-control skills are *active* elements in maintenance; their value lies in continued use, not past successes. Personal science is a lifestyle, not a temporary project. From here on out you should be able to face and conquer new problems with a confidence and background which will make them much more easily surmountable. However, you will never be completely finished with your weight control efforts. If you think so, you're in for trouble. Your life need not be always dominated by dieting, but episodes of difficulty and partial relapse are inevitable. Why?

First, because we live in a world which encourages obesity. Our social customs, the food industry, and our many labor-saving devices invite us to overeat and underexercise. More often than not, the successful reducer is bucking the system in his commendable efforts at self-regulation.

A second factor which will not allow you to rest on your (now thinner) laurels has to do with your biological makeup. You are a perpetually changing organism. It has been estimated that your body's need for food calories decreases by 1 percent each year after age 25. Part of this is because of the increasingly sedentary lifestyle of later years—a pattern which you can now prevent. However, due to the aging process itself, it appears that metabolic requirements generally decline as you get older. This, of course, means that you must be ready to roll with these biological punches—that you must be prepared to adjust your eating and exercise patterns to your ever-changing bodily needs.

All of this is not intended to paint a dismal picture of your future as a weight watcher. We firmly believe that your personal scientist skills have prepared you very well for the task ahead. Relative to any other contemporary approach, you should now be in the best possible position to effect permanent maintenance and lifelong success in the battle of the bulge. We therefore feel that your future will be positive and your efforts well worth their pursuit. Not only are you now optimally prepared for lifelong maintenance, but the entire enterprise should take on a more enjoyable hue. Your weight may have already become a less critical daily theme in your life. With your past progress and growing self-confidence, you need no longer be anxiously obsessed with your daily diet or the uncertainties of your improvement.

As long as you maintain the active, coping perspective of a personal scientist, you can be assured of permanent success. As noted above, occasional difficulties are inevitable—they are a part of life itself. Do not allow these few episodes to throw you into a tailspin of frustration, depression, or resignation. Tell yourself right now that they *will* crop up—and with equal certainty, that you *will* master them. Again, these words of warning should be read with optimism, not panic. For some of you, the inevitability of problems and the endless process of personal science may seem like a rude awakening. It is our opinion, however, that the complacent belief that you have won the battle once and for all invites an even more rude and painful awakening. There should be nothing depressing about the realization that obesity—like many other aspects of life—is a complex problem which can be successfully conquered by a continuing and comfortable life-style of personal science. Relative to thousands of other dieters in the country, your chances of continued progress and enduring improvement are extremely good.

By way of strengthening your preparation even further, we offer the following general guidelines for maintenance and troubleshooting.

1. *When you approach your own chosen level of maintenance, gradually fade out your reliance on structured personal experiments.* That is, try to continue your appropriate eating and activity patterns without requiring some of the former mechanical aspects such as daily self-monitoring. This does not mean to eliminate personal science from your life. Rather, it means that you should be gradually working toward a time when your habits are sufficiently adaptive and comfortable that they no longer need special attention. Note that the transition should be gradual, not abrupt. Also, if you enjoy the structure or support of certain personal science strategies (e.g., recording the intake of problem foods), by all means continue them.

2. *Weigh yourself monthly, chart it, and watch for trends.* If there is one particular date on which you pay bills, turn the calendar, or whatever, make this your monthly checkup. We recommend that it be your only weigh-in, but allow your personal data (not your prejudices) to be the final judge. After your weigh-in, chart your weight so that you can watch for problem trends. If you start to creep in an undesired direction, don your personal scientist lab coat and do a little research. It may be helpful to reread sections of the book dealing with suspected sources of difficulty.

3. *Once per month, evaluate your physical, social, and private environments.* This can easily be done on the same day as your monthly weigh-in. At the bottom of your chart, rate each of your three environments. Are any of them deteriorating toward a fat-enhancing status? If you have previously participated in a group devoted to personal science, why not have a get-together every month or two to maintain support and share problem-solving skills?

4. *Maintain a creative variety in your efforts.* Many dieters report that their failures were often due to boredom or stagnation. Don't allow your reduction or maintenance efforts to go stale. Experiment with new techniques, different foods, and alternate ways of being physically active. This variety will not only make your efforts more enjoyable, but it will also help to develop your flexibility for facing new problems.

5. ***Be prepared for plateaus and problems.*** As stated earlier, occasional episodes of difficulty are inevitable. At this stage of the game, however, they should be more readily handled by your improved technical skills. You can also reduce their difficulty by anticipating them. For example, how might you prepare yourself for a holiday visit or a vacation? What could you do before these events to make room for some desserts or to prepare yourself for negative social feedback? If surgery or childbirth is in your near future, what might you do ahead of time to protect your nutrition without jeopardizing your weight loss progress? If you find yourself becoming disappointed with the rate or amount of your progress, where would you begin to problem solve?

The above recommendations are, of course, extensions of the personal science philosophy. They convey an ongoing commitment to individual growth and active personal responsibility. It has been our experience that this orientation often spills over into other aspects of a person's life. The weight watcher may find that his or her newly acquired skills have additional relevance for improving and enriching other life patterns. And herein, perhaps, lies some of their unique value, for the skills of personal science afford one some very versatile means for achieving many different ends. They are an invaluable avenue to self-regulated growth—a process which, in our opinion, is more accurately portrayed as a journey than a destination. We wish you a thin and happy voyage.

Resource Index

For any given topic, consult the references suggested. Since many of these sources are relatively technical, those containing more practical information for the weight watcher are italicized.

PROCESSES IN OBESITY AND ENERGY METABOLISM
6, 7, 18, 19, 20, 21, 23, 25, 28, 35, 36, 46, 48, 53, 63, 64, 70, 71, 75, 87, 88, 98, *99*, 100, 106, 107, 108, 109, 111, 112, 116, 117, 119, 121, 123, 125, *129*, 132, 133, 134, *136*, 138, *144*, 145, 148, *151*, 152, 154, 155, 156, 157.

HEALTH RISKS IN OBESITY
1, 2, *16, 67*, 92, *99, 129, 143, 144, 151*.

NUTRITION AND DIETETICS
5, 11, 14, 29, 36, *47, 52, 54, 55*, 72, 73, 74, 86, *99, 105*, 118, *129, 143*, 147, 150, *158, 159*.

PRINCIPLES OF SELF-CONTROL
10, 49, 66, 79, 80, 82, 83, 84, 86, *91*, 101, *139*.

EXERCISE
18, 23, *24*, 27, 60, *67*, 78, 92, 97, *99*, 122, *129, 136, 144*.

RESEARCH ON THE TREATMENT OF OBESITY
3, 4, 8, 9, 12, 13, 15, 17, 22, 26, 30, 31, 32, 33, 34, 37, 38, 39, 40, 41, 42, 43, 44, 45, 50, 51, 56, 57, 58, 59, 61, 62, 65, 68, 69, 76, 77, 80, 84, 85, 89, 90, 93, 94, 95, 96, 102, 103, 104, 110, 113, 114, 115, 120, 124, 126, 127, 128, *129*, 130, *131*, 135, *136, 137*, 140, 141, 142, 146, 149, 153.

References

1. Abraham, S.; Collins, G.; and Nordsieck, M. "Relationships of Childhood Weight Status to Morbidity in Adults." *HSMA Health Reports* 86 (1971): 273–284.
2. _____, and Nordsieck, M. "Relationships of Excess Weight in Children and Adults." *Public Health Reports* 75 (1960): 263–273.
3. Abrahms, J. L., and Allen, G. J. "Comparative Effectiveness of Situational Programming, Financial Pay-offs, and Group Pressure in Weight Reduction." *Behavior Therapy* 5 (1974): 391–400.
4. Abramson, E. E. "A Review of Behavioral Approaches to Weight Control." *Behaviour Research and Therapy* 11 (1973): 547–556.
5. Ald, R. *The Skinnylook Cookbook*. New York: New American Library, 1970.
6. Allen, T. H., et. al. "Prediction of Total Adiposity from Skinfolds and the Curvilinear Relationship between External and Internal Adiposity." *Metabolism* 5 (1956): 346–352.
7. Balagura, S. *Hunger: A Biopsychological Analysis*. New York: Basic Books, 1973.
8. Balch, P., and Ross, A. W. "A Behaviorally Oriented Didactic Group Treatment of Obesity: An Exploratory Study." *Journal of Behavior Therapy and Experimental Psychiatry* 5 (1974): 239–243.
9. Balters, H. L. "The Effects of Age of Obesity Onset, Aversive and Non-aversive Weight Reudction Techniques, and Length of Instruction Time on Weight Reduction Measures." Doctoral dissertation, University of Nebraska, 1974.
10. Bandura, A. "Vicarious and Self-reinforcement Processes." In *The Nature of Reinforcement*, edited by R. Glaser, pp. 228–278. New York: Academic Press, 1971.
11. Belinkie, H. *The New Gourmet in the Low-Calorie Kitchen Cookbook*. New York: Avon Publishers, 1971.
12. Bellack, A. S.; Rozensky, R.; and Schwartz, J. "A Comparison of Two Forms of Self-monitoring in a Behavioral Weight Reduction Program." *Behavior Therapy* 5 (1974): 523–530.
13. _____; Schwartz, J.; and Rozensky, R. H. "The Contribution of External Control to Self-control in a Weight Reduction Program." *Journal of Behavior Therapy and Experimental Psychiatry* 5 (1974): 245–249.
14. Berland, T. *Rating the Diets*. Skokie, Ill.: Consumer Guide, 1974.
15. Bernard, J. L. "Rapid Treatment of Gross Obesity by Operant Techniques." *Psychological Reports* 23 (1968): 663–666.

16. Blumenfeld, A. *Heart Attack: Are You a Candidate?* New York: Pyramid, 1964.

17. Bornstein, P. H., and Sipprelle, C. N. "Group Treatment of Obesity by Induced Anxiety." *Behaviour Research and Therapy* 11 (1973): 339–341.

18. Bradfield, R. B., and Jourdan, M. "Energy Expenditure of Obese Women during Weight Loss." *American Journal of Clinical Nutrition* 25 (1972): 971–975.

19. Bray, G. A. "Effect of Caloric Restriction on Energy Expenditure in Obese Patients." *Lancet* 2 (1969): 397.

20. Bruch, H. *Eating Disorders: Obesity, Anorexia Nervosa, and the Person Within.* New York: Basic Books, 1973.

21. Campbell, R.; Hashim, S. A.; and Van Itallie, T. B. "Studies of Food Intake Regulation in Man." *New England Journal of Medicine* 285 (1972): 1402–1407.

22. Cautela, J. R. "Treatment of Compulsive Behavior by Covert Sensitization." *Psychological Record* 16 (1966): 33–41.

23. Chirico, A. M., and Stunkard, A. J. "Physical Activity and Human Obesity." *New England Journal of Medicine* 263 (1960): 935–946.

24. Cooper, K. H. *The New Aerobics.* New York: M. Evans & Co., 1970.

25. Davenport, C. B. *Body Build and Its Inheritance.* Carnegie Institute of Washington, Publication No. 329, 1923.

26. Dinoff, M.; Rickard, H. C.; and Colwick, J. "Weight Reduction through Successive Contracts." *American Journal of Orthopsychiatry* 42 (1972): 110–113.

27. Durnin, J. V. G. A., and Passmore, R. *Energy, Work and Leisure.* London: Heinemann Educational Books, 1967.

28. _____, and Rahaman, M. M. "The Assessment of Amount of Fat in the Human Body from Measurements of Skinfold Thickness." *British Journal of Nutrition* 21 (1967): 681–689.

29. Ewald, E. B. *Recipes for a Small Planet.* New York: Ballantine, 1973.

30. Fernan, W. "The Role of Experimenter Contact in Behavioral Bibliotherapy of Obesity." Master's thesis, Pennsylvania State University, 1973.

31. Ferster, C. B.; Nurnbeger, J. I.; and Levitt, E. B. "The Control of Eating." *Journal of Mathetics* 1 (1962): 87–109.

32. Finkelstein, B., and Fryer, B. A. "Meal Frequency and Weight Reduction of Young Women." *American Journal of Clinical Nutrition* 24 (1971): 465–468.

33. Foreyt, J. P., and Hagen, R. L. "Covert Sensitization: Conditioning or Suggestion?" *Journal of Abnormal Psychology* 82 (1973): 17–23.

34. _____, and Kennedy, W. A. "Treatment of Overweight by Aversion Therapy." *Behaviour Research and Therapy* 9 (1971): 29–34.

35. Gaul, D. J.; Craighead, W. E.; and Mahoney, M. J. "The Relationship between Eating Rates and Obesity." *Journal of Consulting and Clinical Psychology* 43 (1975): 123–125.

36. Guyton, A. C. *Textbook of Medical Physiology.* Philadelphia: W. B. Saunders, 1971.

37. Hagen, R. L. "Group Therapy versus Bibliotherapy in Weight Reduction." *Behavior Therapy* 5 (1974): 222–234.

38. Hall, S. M. "Self-control and Therapist Control in the Behavioral Treatment of Overweight Women." *Behaviour Research and Therapy* 10 (1972): 59–68.

39. _____. "Behavior Treatment of Obesity: A Two-year Follow-up." *Behaviour Research and Therapy* 11 (1973): 647–748.

40. _____, and Hall, R. G. "Outcome and Methodological Considerations in Behavioral Treatment of Obesity." *Behavior Therapy* 5 (1974): 352–364.

41. _____; _____; Hanson, R. W.; and Bordon, B. L. "Permanence of Two Self-managed Treatments of Overweight in University and Community Populations." *Journal of Consulting and Clinical Psychology* 42 (1974): 781–786.

42. Harmatz, M. G., and Lapuc, P. "Behavior Modification of Overeating in a Psychiatric Population." *Journal of Consulting and Clinical Psychology* 32 (1968): 583–587.

43. Harris, M. B. "Self-directed Program for Weight Control: A Pilot Study." *Journal of Abnormal Psychology* 74 (1969): 263–270.

44. _____, and Bruner, C. G. "A Comparison of a Self-control and a Contract Procedure for Weight Control." *Behaviour Research and Therapy* 9 (1971): 347–354.

45. _____, and Hallbauer, E. S. "Self-directed Weight Control through Eating and Exercise." *Behaviour Research and Therapy* 11 (1973): 523–529.

46. Hashim, S. A., and Van Itallic, T. B. "Studies in Normal and Obese Subjects Using a Monitored Food-dispensing Device." *Annals of the New York Academy of Science* 131 (1965): 654–661.

47. Heiss, K. B., and Heiss, C. G. *Eat to Your Heart's Content: The Low Cholesterol Gourmet Cookbook.* New York: New American Library, 1972.

48. Hirsch, J., and Knittle, J. L. "Cellularity of Obese and Nonobese Human Adipose Tissue." *Federation Proceedings* 29 (1971): 1516–1521.

49. Homme, L. E. "Perspectives in Psychology: XXIV. Control of Coverants, the Operants of the Mind." *Psychological Record* 15 (1965): 501–511.

50. Horan, J. J.; Baker, S. B.; Hoffman, A. M.; and Shute, R. E. "Weight Loss through Variations in the Coverant Control Paradigm." *Journal of Consulting and Clinical Psychology* 43 (1975): 68–72.

51. _____, and Johnson, R. G. "Coverant Conditioning through a Self-management Application of the Premack Principle: Its Effect on Weight Reduction." *Journal of Behavior Therapy and Experimental Psychiatry* 2 (1971): 243–249.

52. Hunter, B. T. *Consumer Beware.* New York: Simon & Schuster, 1971.

53. Jacobs, J. L., and Sharma, K. N. "Taste versus Calories: Sensory and Metabolic Signals in the Control of Food Intake." *Annals of the New York Academy of Science* 157 (1969): 1084–1125.

54. Jacobson, M. F. *Eater's Digest.* Garden City, N.Y.: Doubleday, 1972.

55. _____. *Nutrition Scoreboard.* Washington, D.C.: Center for Science in the Public Interest, 1973.

56. Janda, L. H., and Rimm, D. C. "Covert Sensitization in the Treatment of Obesity." *Journal of Abnormal Psychology* 80 (1972): 37–42.

57. Jeffrey, D. B. "Self-control versus External Control in the Modification and Maintenance of Weight Loss." In *Applications of Behavior Therapy to Health Care,* edited by R. C. Katz and S. I. Aluntnick. New York: Pergamon, forthcoming.

58. _____, and Christensen, E. R. "The Relative Efficacy of Behavior Therapy, Will Power, and No-treatment Control Procedures for Weight Loss." Paper read at the Sixth Annual Meeting of the Association for the Advancement of Behavior Therapy, October 1972, New York, N.Y.

59. _____; _____; and Pappas, J. P. "A Case Study Report of a Behavioral Modification Weight Reduction Group: Treatment and Follow-up." Paper read at the Rocky Mountain Psychological Association, 1972, Albuquerque, N.M.

60. Johnson, M. L.; Burke, B. S.; and Mayer, J. "Relative Importance of Inactivity and Overeating in the Energy Balance of Obese High School Girls." *American Journal of Clinical Nutrition* 4 (1956): 37–44.

61. Jongmans, J. G. "Vermagerings-Therapieen." Doctoral dissertation, Psychological Laboratory of the University of Amsterdam, 1969.

62. _____. "Een ontwerp voor een vermageringsmodel." Unpublished manuscript, Psychological Laboratory of the University of Amsterdam, 1970.

63. Jordan, H. A. "Voluntary Intragastric Feeding: Oral and Gastric Contribution to Food Intake and Hunger in Man." *Journal of Comparative Physiological Psychology* 68 (1969): 498–506.

64. _____. "Physiological Control of Food Intake in Man." Paper read at the Fogarty International Conference on Obesity, October 1973, Washington, D.C.

65. _____, and Levitz, L. S. "A Behavioral Approach to the Problem of Obesity." In *Obesity: Pathogenesis and Management,* edited by T. Silverstone and J. Fincham. Lancaster: Medical and Technical Publishing Co., 1975.

66. Kazdin, A. E. "Self-monitoring and Behavior Change." In *Self-control: Power to the Person,* edited by M. J. Mahoney and C. E. Thoresen. Monterey: Brooks/Cole, 1974.

67. Kannel, W. B. "The Disease of Living." *Nutrition Today* 6 (1971): 2–11.

68. Kennedy, W. A., and Foreyt, J. "Control of Eating Behavior in an Obese Patient by Avoidance Conditioning." *Psychological Reports* 22 (1968): 571–576.

69. Kerbauy, R. R. "Autocontrole: Manipulacao de condicoes antecedentes e consequentes do compartamento alimentar." Doctoral dissertation, University of São Paulo, Brazil, 1972.

70. Keys, A.; Brozek, J.; Henschel, A.; Mickelson, O.; and Taylor, H. L. *The Biology of Human Starvation.* 2 vols. Minneapolis: University of Minnesota Press, 1950.

71. Knittle, J. L., and Hirsch, J. "Effect of Early Nutrition on the Development of the Rat Epididymal Fat Pads: Cellularity and Metabolism." *Journal of Clinical Investigation* 47 (1968): 2091–2098.

72. Lappé, F. M. *Diet for a Small Planet.* New York: Ballantine, 1971.

73. Lawlor, T., and Wells, D. G. "The Metabolic Hazards of Fasting." *American Journal of Clinical Nutrition* 22 (1969): 1142.

74. Leveille, G. A., and Romsos, D. R. "Meal Eating and Obesity." *Nutrition Today* 9 (1974): 4–9.

75. Levitz, L. S. "The Susceptibility of Human Feeding Behavior to External Control." Paper read at the Fogarty International Conference on Obesity, October 1973, Washington, D.C.

76. _____, and Stunkard, A. J. "Intervening with Behavior Therapy in Self-help Groups for Weight Control: Preliminary Report." Paper read at the Sixth Annual Meeting of the Association for the Advancement of Behavior Therapy, October 1972, New York, N.Y.

77. Lick, J., and Bootzin, R. "Covert Sensitization for the Treatment of Obesity." Paper presented to the Midwestern Psychological Association, 1971, Detroit, Mich.

78. Lincoln, J. E. "Calorie Intake, Obesity, and Physical Activity." *American Journal of Clinical Nutrition* 25 (1972): 390–394.

79. Locke, E. Q.; Cartledge, N.; and Koeppel, J. "Motivational Effects of Knowledge of Results: A Goal-setting Phenomenon?" *Psychological Bulletin* 70 (1968): 474–485.

80. Mahoney, K., and Mahoney, M. J. "Cognitive Factors in Weight Reduction." In *Counseling Methods,* edited by J. D. Krumboltz and C. E. Thoresen. New York: Holt, Rinehart and Winston, 1975.

81. Mahoney, M. J. "Toward an Experimental Analysis of Coverant Control." *Behavior Therapy* 1 (1970): 510–521.

82. _____. "Research Issues in Self-management." *Behavior Therapy* 3 (1972): 45–63.

83. _____. "Self-control Strategies in Weight Loss." Paper read at the Sixth Annual Meeting of the Association for the Advancement of Behavior Therapy, October 1972, New York, N.Y.

84. _____. "Clinical Issues in Self-control Training." Paper read at the American Psychological Association, August 1973, Montreal, Canada.

85. _____. Self-reward and Self-monitoring Techniques for Weight Control." *Behavior Therapy* 5 (1974): 48–57.

86. _____. *Cognition and Behavior Modification.* Cambridge, Mass.: Ballinger, 1974.

87. _____. "Fat Fiction." *Behavior Therapy* 6 (1975), in press.

88. _____. "The Obese Eating Style: Bites, Beliefs, and Behavior Modification." *Addictive Behaviors* 1 (1975), in press.

89. _____, and Mahoney, K. "Treatment of Obesity: A Clinical Exploration." In *Obesity: Behavioral Approaches to Dietary Management,* edited by B. J. Williams, S. Martin, and J. P. Foreyt, New York: Brunner/Mazel, 1976.

90. _____; Moura, N. G. M.; and Wade, T. C. "The Relative Efficacy of Self-reward, Self-punishment, and Self-monitoring Techniques for Weight Loss." *Journal of Consulting and Clinical Psychology* 40 (1973): 404–407.

91. _____, and Thoresen, C. E., eds. *Self-control: Power to the Person.* Monterey, Calif.: Brooks/Cole, 1974.

92. Mann, G. V.; Garrett, H. L.; Farhi, H.; and Billings, F. T. "Exercise and Heart Disease." *American Journal of Medicine* 46 (1969): 12–27.

93. Mann, R. A. "The Behavior-therapeutic Use of Contingency Contracting to Control an Adult Behavior Problem: Weight Control." *Journal of Applied Behavior Analysis* 5 (1972): 99–109.

94. _____. "The Use of Contingency Contracting to Facilitate Durability of Be-

havior Change: Weight Loss Maintenance." Paper read at the American Psychological Association, August 1973, Montreal, Canada.

95. Manno, B., and Marston, A. R. "Weight Reduction as a Function of Negative Covert Reinforcement (Sensitization) versus Positive Covert Reinforcement. *Behaviour Research and Therapy* 10 (1972): 201–207.

96. Martin, J. E., and Sachs, D. A. "The Effects of a Self-control Weight Loss Program on an Obese Woman." *Journal of Behavior Therapy and Experimental Psychiatry* 4 (1973): 155–159.

97. Mayer, J. "Correlation between Metabolism and Feeding Behavior and Multiple Etiology of Obesity." *Bulletin of the New York Academy of Medicine* 22 (1957): 744–761.

98. _____. "Genetic Factors in Obesity." *Annals of the New York Academy of Sciences* 131 (1965): 412–421.

99. _____. *Overweight: Causes, Cost, and Control.* Englewood Cliffs: Prentice-Hall, 1968.

100. _____, and Thomas, D. W. "Regulation of Food Intake and Obesity." *Science* 156 (1967): 328–327.

101. Meichenbaum, D., and Cameron, R. "The Clinical Potential of Modifying What Clients Say to Themselves." In *Self-control: Power to the Person,* edited by M. J. Mahoney and C. E. Thoresen. Monterey: Brooks/Cole, 1974.

102. Meyer, V., and Crisp, A. H. "Aversion Therapy in Two Cases of Obesity." *Behaviour Research and Therapy* 2 (1964): 143–147.

103. Moore, C. H., and Crum, B. C. "Weight Reduction in a Chronic Schizophrenic by Means of Operant Conditioning Procedures: A Case Study." *Behaviour Research and Therapy* 7 (1969): 129–131.

104. Morganstern, K. P. "Cigarette Smoke as a Noxious Stimulus in Self-managed Aversion Therapy for Compulsive Eating." *Behavior Therapy* 5 (1974): 255–260.

105. Netzer, C. *The Brand-name Calorie Counter.* New York: Dell Publishing Co., 1969.

106. Nisbett, R. E. "Determinants of Food Intake in Human Obesity." *Science* 159 (1968): 1254–1255.

107. _____, and Kanouse, D. E. "Obesity, Food Deprivation, and Supermarket Shopping Behavior." *Journal of Personality and Social Psychology* 12 (1969): 289–294.

108. Passmore, R.; Meiklejohn, A. P.; Dewar, A. D.; and Thow, R. K. "Energy Utilization in Overfed Thin Young Men." *British Journal of Nutrition* 9 (1955): 20.

109. _____; Strong, A.; Swindells, Y. E.; and El Din, N. "The Effect of Overfeeding on Two Fat Young Women." *British Journal of Nutrition* 17 (1963): 373.

110. Penick, S. B.; Filion, R.; Fox, S.; and Stunkard, A. J. "Behavior Modification in the Treatment of Obesity." *Psychosomatic Medicine* 33 (1971): 49–55.

111. Polivy, J. "Perception of Calories and Regulation of Intake in Man and Animals." Unpublished manuscript, Loyola University of Chicago, 1975.

112. Rodahl, K., & Issekutz, B., eds. *Fat as a Tissue.* New York: McGraw-Hill, 1964.

113. Romanczyk, R. G. "Self-monitoring in the Treatment of Obesity: Parameters of Reactivity." *Behavior Therapy* 5 (1974): 531–540.

114. _____; Tracey, D. A.; Wilson, G. T.; and Thorpe, G. L. "Behavioral Techniques in the Treatment of Obesity: A Comparative Analysis." *Behaviour Research and Therapy* 11 (1973): 629–640.

115. Sachs, L. B., and Ingram, G. L. "Covert Sensitization as a Treatment for Weight Control." *Psychological Reports* 30 (1972): 971–974.

116. Schachter, S. "Some Extraordinary Facts about Obese Humans and Rats." *American Psychologist* 26 (1971): 129–144.

117. _____, and Rodin, J., eds. *Obese Humans and Rats.* Hillsdale, N.J.: Lawrence Erlbaum Associates, 1974.

118. Schauf, G. E. "All Calories Don't Count . . . Perhaps." *Nutrition Today,* September-October 1971, p. 16.

119. Seltzer, C. C., and Mayer, J. "Body Build and Obesity—Who Are the Obese?" *Journal of the American Medical Association* 189 (1964): 677–684.

120. Shipman, W. "Behavior Therapy with Obese Dieters." *Annual Report of the Institute for Psychosomatic and Psychiatric Research and Training,* pp. 70–71. Chicago: Michael Reese Hospital and Medical Center. 1970.

121. Sims, E. A.; Goldman, R. F.; Gluck, C. M.; Horton, E. S.; Kellerher, P. C.; and Rowe, D. W. "Experimental Obesity in Man." *Transactions of the Association of American Physicians* 81 (1968): 153–170.

122. Soule, R. G., and Goldman, R. F. "Energy Costs of Loads Carried on the Head, Hands, or Feet." *Journal of Applied Physiology* 27 (1969): 687–690.

123. Spiegel, T. A. "Caloric Regulation of Food Intake in Man." *Journal of Comparative Psychology* 84 (1973): 24–37.

124. Steffy, R. A. "Service Applications: Psychotic Adolescents and Adults." Paper read at the American Psychological Association, September 1968, San Francisco, Calif.

125. Stellar, E. "Hunger in Man: Comparative and Physiological Studies." *American Psychologist* 22 (1967): 105–117.

126. Stollak, G. E. "Weight Loss Obtained under Different Experimental Procedures." *Psychotherapy: Theory, Research and Practice* 4 (1967): 61–64.

127. Stuart, R. B. "Behavioral Control of Overeating." *Behaviour Research and Therapy* 5 (1967): 357–365.

128. _____. "A Three-dimensional Program for the Treatment of Obesity." *Behaviour Research and Therapy* 9 (1971): 177–186.

129. _____, and Davis, B. *Slim Chance in a Fat World: Behavioral Control of Obesity.* Champaign, Illinois: Research Press, 1972.

130. Stunkard, A. J. "The Management of Obesity." *New York Journal of Medicine,* 58 (1958): 79–87.

131. _____. "New Therapies for the Eating Disorders: Behavior Modification of Obesity and Anorexia Nervosa." *Archives of General Psychiatry* 26 (1972): 391–398.

132. _____. "Anorexia Nervosa." In *The Science and Practice of Clinical Medicine,* edited by J. P. Sanford. New York: Grune & Stratton, forthcoming.

133. _____, and Burt, V. "Obesity and the Body Image: II. Age at Onset of Dis-

turbances in the Body Image." *American Journal of Psychiatry* 123 (1967): 1443–1447.

134. _____, and Fox, S. "The Relationship of Gastric Motility and Hunger: A Summary of the Evidence." *Psychosomatic Medicine* 33 (1971): 123–134.

135. _____; Levine, H.; and Fox, S. "The Management of Obesity: Patient Self-help and Medical Treatment." *Archives of Internal Medicine* 125 (1970): 1067–1072.

136. _____, and Mahoney, M. J. "Hope for the Obese: Behavior Modification." In *Psychiatry,* edited by E. Robins, pp. 45–53. New York: McGraw-Hill, 1972.

137. _____, and _____. "Behavioral Treatment of the Eating Disorders." In *Handbook of Behavior Modification,* edited by H. Leitenberg. Englewood Cliffs, N.J.: Prentice-Hall, 1976.

138. Tabas, L., and Jordan, H. A. "Ingestive Behavior of Obese and Thin Humans Eating in a Restaurant." Unpublished manuscript, University of Pennsylvania, 1973.

139. Thoresen, C. E., and Mahoney, M. J. *Behavioral Self-control.* New York: Holt, Rinehart and Winston, 1974.

140. Thorpe, J. G.; Schmidt, E.; Brown, P. T.; and Castell, D. "Aversion-relief Therapy: A New Method for General Application." *Behaviour Research and Therapy* 2 (1964): 71–82.

141. Tyler, V. O., and Straughan, J. H. "Coverant Control and Breath Holding as Techniques for the Treatment of Obesity." *Psychological Record* 20 (1970): 473–478.

142. Upper, D., and Newton, J. G. "A Weight-reduction Program for Schizophrenic Patients on a Token Economy Unit: Two Case Studies." *Journal of Behavior Therapy and Experimental Psychiatry* 2 (1971): 113–115.

143. U. S. Department of Agriculture. *Food and Your Health.* Publication No. 547. Washington, D.C.: U. S. Government Printing Office, 1969.

144. U. S. Public Health Service. *Obesity and Health.* Publication No. 1485. Washington, D.C.: U. S. Government Printing Office, 1966.

145. Walike, B. C.; Jordan, H. A.; and Stellar, E. "Preloading and the Regulation of Food Intake in Man." *Journal of Comparative and Physiological Psychology* 68 (1969): 327–333.

146. Weisenberg, M., and Fray, E. "What's Missing in the Treatment of Obesity by Behavior Modification?" *Journal of the American Dietetic Association* 65 (1974): 410–414.

147. Welles, S. L. "Nutritive Intake of Members of Weight Reduction Programs." Master's thesis, Pennsylvania State University, 1973.

148. Wiepkema, P. R. "Behavioral Factors in the Regulation of Food Intake." *Proceedings of the Nutrition Society* 30 (1971): 142–149.

149. Wijesinghe, B. "Massed Electrical Aversion Treatment of Compulsive Eating." *Journal of Behavior Therapy and Experimental Psychiatry* 4 (1973): 133–135.

150. Williams, S. R. *Nutrition and Diet Therapy.* St. Louis: C. V. Mosby, 1973.

151. Winick, M. "Childhood Obesity." *Nutrition Today* 9 (1974): 6–12.

152. Withers, R. F. L. "Problems in the Genetics of Human Obesity." *Eugenics Review* 56 (1964): 81–90.

153. Wollersheim, J. P. "The Effectiveness of Group Therapy Based upon Learning Principles in the Treatment of Overweight Women." *Journal of Abnormal Psychology* 76 (1970): 462–474.
154. Wooley, O. W. "Long-term Food Regulation in the Obese and Nonobese." *Psychosomatic Medicine* 33 (1971): 436–444.
155. _____, and Wooley, S. C. "The Experimental Psychology of Obesity." In *Obesity: Pathogenesis and Management,* edited by T. Silverstone and J. Fincham. Lancaster: Medical and Technical Publishing Company, 1975.
156. _____; _____; and Dunham, R. B. "Can Calories Be Perceived and Do They Affect Hunger in Obese and Nonobese Humans?" *Journal of Comparative and Physiological Psychology* 80 (1972): 250–258.
157. Wooley, S. C. "Physiologic versus Cognitive Factors in Short-term Food Regulation in the Obese and Nonobese." *Psychosomatic Medicine* 34 (1972): 62–68.
158. Young, C. M. "Planning the Low Calorie Diet." *American Journal of Clinical Nutrition* 8 (1960): 896–900.
159. Yudkin, J. *Sweet and Dangerous.* New York: Bantam, 1972.